PHARMACEUTICAL CALCULATIONS

A MANUAL FOR STUDENTS AND PRACTITIONERS

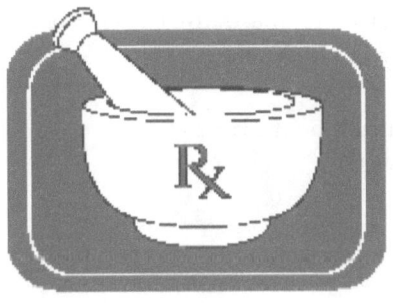

Willbrord Maddo Kalala (PhD)

B Pharm, M Sc Pharm

Copyright © 2016 by Willbrord Maddo Kalala (PhD).

Library of Congress Control Number:		2016906789
ISBN:	Hardcover	978-1-5144-8871-3
	Softcover	978-1-5144-8870-6
	eBook	978-1-5144-8869-0

All rights reserved. No part of this book may be reproduced or transmitted in any form or by any means, electronic or mechanical, including photocopying, recording, or by any information storage and retrieval system, without permission in writing from the copyright owner.

Any people depicted in stock imagery provided by Thinkstock are models, and such images are being used for illustrative purposes only.
Certain stock imagery © Thinkstock.

Print information available on the last page.

Rev. date: 10/11/2018

To order additional copies of this book, contact:
Xlibris
1-888-795-4274
www.Xlibris.com
Orders@Xlibris.com
740929

CONTENTS

TABLE OF CONTENTS	3
Preface	5
Introduction	6
Chapter 1 Review of Basic Mathematics	7
Chapter 2 Interpretation of Prescriptions	25
Chapter 3 Weights and Measures	31
Chapter 4 Computations in Metric Systems	41
Chapter 5 Apothecary and Avoirdupois Systems Compared to Metric System	44
Chapter 6 Conversion of Metric/Common/Metric Systems	49
Chapter 7 Calculations involving Density and Specific Gravity	53
Chapter 8 Calculation of Doses	57
Chapter 9 Expression of Concentrations in Pharmaceutical Preparations	71
Chapter 10 Calculations involving formulations: enlarging and Reducing Formulae	85
Chapter 11 Dilutions and Concentrations	87
Chapter 12 Expression of Concentration of Electrolytes: Milliequivalents Millimoles and milliosmoles	116
Chapter 13 Isotonic Solutions	126
Chapter 14 Thermometry	141
Chapter 15 Calculations Involving Intravenous Nutritional Supplimentation	144
Chapter 16 Worked Examples	153
Chapter 17 Practice Questions	160

"The pharmacy calculations manual has been presented in a very simple and easy to follow manner, enriched with a lot of worked examples, which makes it easy to follow even for students lacking good mathematics foundation"

S.S. Senya, Former Principle of the School of Pharmaceutical Sciences, and Director of the Institute of Allied Health Sciences, Muhimbili University of Health and Allied Sciences. Also a long term tutor in Pharmaceutical calculations.

PREFACE

The pharmaceutical sector is rapidly growing globally, and this has resulted in the increased demand of personnel. To meet this demand, there are several colleges that train pharmacy profession at various levels, that is Certificate, Diploma and Degree levels. There are also other colleges that train related professions that deal deal with pharmaceuticals including nurse students and prospective clinical officers. A student in any of these colleges is moulded academically to be proficient in the profession. Students are trained in bodily functions (Anatomy, physiology, biochemistry and other basic sciences) and pharmaceutical core subjects (pharmaceutics, pharmacology, microbiology, pharmacognosy and medicinal chemistry). Bofore a student graduates he/she must be able to prepare medicines extemporaneously (at the bench on small scale) or at industrial large scale level. In all cases, a thorough knowledge of mathematics is paramount to be able to calculate properly the required amounts of ingredients to prepare medicines and reagents (i.e. Compounding and Dispensing). They must be able also to determine appropriate doses in children and adults, and estimating appropriate quantites of medicines required in compromised patients such as in kidney or liver failure. Hence the mastery of pharmaceutical calculations.

There are many textbooks in Pharmaceutical Calculations. But having tought pharmaceutical calculations at the University level for the past 25 years. I came to realize that our students face various problems. First of all, they come from various backgrounds. Some students are good in mathematics, but some lack the proper background hence are not as good. I have designed this manual to simply provide a reference material in pharmaceutical calculations that can be used by students of all levels (dispensers, pharmaceutical assistants and technicians as well as pharmacy degree students) regardless of their backgrounds. The manual addresses both situations by helping the few tutors available to help students understand practical problems that occur in practice from time to time. In writing this manual, I followed the various curricula of pharmacy at certificate, diploma and degree levels of various institutions. The manual also addresses components of the curriculum of Nursing courses, particularly calculations involving doses and dosages. Thus trainers will choose topics relevant to the level they are dealing with.

The simplicity with which the material is presented is designed to help students to be able to study by themselves even in the absence of tutors. It is enriched with over 350 worked examples and about 150 practice questions with answers to make self-study possible. With many practical worked examples, even the slowest learner can be taken on board. Furthermore, this manual will be a quick reference for practicing pharmaceutical technicians, nurses and pharmacists.

The first chapter reviews and introduces the reader to the basics of mathematics. Whereas these are expected to be understood by pharmacy students, some students may have forgotten them but some students may not be conversant with some of them at all. It is important for trainers to ensure that all students are conversant with the basics of mathematics before attempting to proceed with the rest of the manual.

Willbrord Kalala,
Lecturer, School of Pharmacy, Muhimbili University of Health and Allied Sciences.

INTRODUCTION

The practice of pharmacy requires knowledge in basic mathematics to perform every day jobs. Pharmacists, pharmaceutical technicians, Assistants and dispensers need to interpret orders, dispense medication and perform pharmaceutical calculations. The mathematics used covers basic arithmetic; fractions and decimals; Roman numerals; percentages; systems of measurements; ratios and proportions, and basic algebra.

When filling prescriptions and tracking inventory, one employs addition, subtraction, multiplication and division. Many dosage calculations use amounts other than whole numbers. Mathematics is needed to compute operations such as dosage conversions, Intravenous admixtures and administration of drug dose over time. Therefore, one must be able to add, subtract, multiply and divide fractions. One must be able to understand decimals and place values, as converting fractions to decimals and decimals into fractions is not uncommon.

Roman numerals are still used by some physicians in dosage computations. We must be able to interpret these computations correctly.

Although we use metric system for weights and measures, occasionally we may encounter different systems of measurement, such as the avoirdupois system, the apothecary system, and household measurements. We must be able to identify and understand units from each system and be able to convert amounts from one system to the next.

Pharmaceutical calculations and conversions require the use of ratios, proportions and percentages. You may be called upon to convert fractions to ratios and vice versa. You may also need to convert percentages to fractions or decimals and vice versa.

When performing a pharmaceutical calculation, one often is required to solve for an unknown quantity. We use basic algebra to do this. Most commonly, the algebra is combined with proportions and percentages in order to calculate a new amount.

Many problems can be solved by more than one procedure or method. Any logical method that gives the correct answer is allowed, provided you get the correct answer. Thus the solutions to sample problems given here are among possible solutions rather than the only way to tackle the problems. The best way is the one that is understood clearly and which leads to correct answer.

When presented with a problem, read carefully, whether it is a prescription, chart, order, formula, table etc., in order to identify the necessary data and information given.

- Identify the required information
- Place decimal places correctly – many errors are due to carelessness such as decimal point placement
- Logically tackle the problem
- Several steps may be necessary. Don't use shortcuts unless you are very certain.
- Put all measurements in one system and expression e.g. SI units Kg, g, mL, L, % ratio strength.

CHAPTER 1

REVIEW OF BASIC MATHEMATICS

This Review is designed to familiarize you with the mathematical skills and concepts that are needed to solve pharmaceutical calculations in compounding and dispensing. It includes arithmetic and algebra with worked examples and there is a set of exercises (with answers) at the end of each section. This review is not intended to be comprehensive. It is assumed that certain basic concepts are common knowledge to all students and prospective users of this manual. Emphasis is therefore placed on the more important skills, concepts, and definitions, and on those particular areas that are frequently confused or misunderstood. If any of the topics seem especially unfamiliar, we encourage you to consult appropriate mathematics text books for a more detailed treatment of those topics.

1.1 THE BASICS OF CALCULATIONS

Most of the problems you will be dealing with will involve Addition, Subtraction, Multiplication and Division. Moreover, you may be required to convert one system of measurement or weighing into the other or one type of units into the other. Either way, you will need to use one or more of such manipulations. Whereas we believe that prior to joining the course of pharmacy you did some mathematics, let us take time to review rules governing these basic manipulations.

If you come across a problem involving Addition, Subtraction, Multiplication or Division, here are important rules to follow:

1.1.1 Addition

Add like quantities. You cannot for example add kilograms, milligrams and liters together. Add similar units and if necessary convert to common units

Q1. Add 5kg, 45grams and 454milligrams	First of all, convert to common units: 5kg　　　　　　= 5 x 1000 grams = 5000.0 g 45 grams　　　 =　　　　　　　　　45 .0 g 454 milligrams = 454g ÷ 1000 =　　0. 454 g 　　　　　　　　　　　　　　　　5045.454 g
Q2. Add 78.98, 0.004, 342.7 and 3.5	When adding decimals keep the decimal points directly under each other: 　　78.98 　　 0.004 　　342.7 +　　 3.5 　　425.184

When adding fractions reduce to the lowest common denominator, add the resulting numerators and reduce the fraction if possible by cancelling.

Q3.	$\frac{2}{3}+\frac{4}{5}+\frac{1}{6}+\frac{1}{4}$	The common denominator is obtained by multiplying all the denominators: $3x5x6x4 = 360$. Each numerator is found by multiplying the fraction by the common denominator: i) $\frac{2}{3}$ x 360 = 240 ii) $\frac{4}{5}x360 = 288$ iii) $\frac{1}{6}x360 = 60$ iv) $\frac{1}{4}x360 = 80$ Thus $\frac{2}{3}+\frac{4}{5}+\frac{1}{6}+\frac{1}{4} = \frac{240+288+60+80}{360}$ $= \frac{668}{360}$ $= \frac{167}{90}$ $= 1\frac{77}{90}$ Answer
Q4.	$\frac{1}{4}+\frac{1}{2}+\frac{3}{8}$	$= \frac{2+4+3}{8} = \frac{9}{8}$ $= 1\frac{1}{9}$ Answer

1.1.2. Subtraction

Subtract only like quantities. If the quantities are not alike, change them to common units.

Q5. How much is left in a container previously containing 5 liters of alcohol after withdrawal of 60 mL, 2 liters and 2.22 centiliters?	First get the total volume withdrawn: 60mL +2 liters+2.22 centiliters = 60mL +2000 mL+22.2 mL = 2082.2 mL Then convert to like units and subtract: 5 liters = 5 x 1000 mL = 5000 mL 2082.2 Milliliters = 2082.2 mL Amount remaining = 2917.8 mL Ans.

1.1.3. Multiplication

The product has the same denomination as the multiplicand.

Q6. Multiply 56 .1 mL by 12	$56.1x12 = 673.2\ mL$
Q7. How many milligrams are used to make 1200 units, each of which contains 250 µg of a drug?	$1200 \times 250 = 300000\ µg = 300\ mg$

If the multiplicand is composed of different denominations change to common unit before multiplying and reduce the product to measurable units.

Q8. We have two sets of bottles containing medicines. The first set has three bottles each of which containing 900 mg of the medicine, and the second set consists of four bottles each having 1.5 g of the medicine. What is the weight of the total medicine in all seven bottles?	Total weight: first set = 3 x 900mg = 2700 mg Second set = 4 x 1.5 g = 6.0 g = <u>6000 mg</u> Total weight = 8700 mg or 8.7 g

Multiply fractions and decimals in any arithmetic problem and reduce quantities to measurable of weighable units.

Q9. You are required to prepare Five liters of a solution of clindamycin containing 650.5 mg of clindamycin per mL. How many grams of clindamycin are required?	650.5 mg x 5 (liters) x 1000 mL/liter = 3252500mg = 3252.5 grams
Q10. How many meters can you make if you join six poles each having ¾ meter?	$\frac{3}{4} \times 6 = \frac{18}{4} = 4\frac{2}{4} = 4\frac{1}{2}$ meters

1.1.4. Division

The quotient always has the same denominations as the dividend

Q11. If you had 5 liters of juice and give equal amount to 6 of you friends, what volume would each of them get?	$\frac{5L}{6} = 0.83\ liter$ or $833\ mL$

If there are different denominations, make a common unit and treat fractions and decimals just like in multiplication.

Q12. The dose of a drug is 250 mg. How many doses can we have from 2 kilograms of the drug?	2 kilograms = 2000 grams = 2000000 mg. Therefore, we can get $\frac{2000000}{250} = 8000\ doses$

1.2 ARITHMETIC

We would like to remind you some rules for performing basic arithmetic operations with integers, which we assume are familiar to you, but you, may have forgotten.

(i) Multiplication by 0 always results in 0		e.g., 0 x 23 = 0.
(ii) Division by 0 is not defined		e.g., 8 ÷ 0 has no meaning.
(iii) Multiplication (or division) of two integers with different signs yields a negative result.	e.g., -4 x 12 = - 48.	-16 ÷ 4 = -4.

(iv) Multiplication (or division) of two *negative* integers yields a positive result	e.g., $-3 \times -5 = 15$ and $-32 \div -8 = 4$.
The division of one integer by another yields either a zero remainder, sometimes called *"dividing evenly,"* or a positive-integer remainder. (v) If an integer N is *divisible by* an integer x, it means that N divided by x yields a zero remainder.	$\begin{array}{r}43\\5\overline{)215}\\\underline{20}\\15\\\underline{15}\\0 = \text{no reminder}\end{array}$ $\quad\quad\begin{array}{r}2\\13\overline{)36}\\\underline{26}\\10 = \text{Reminder}\end{array}$
(vi) The multiplication of two integers yields a third integer. The first two integers are called *factors*, and the third integer is called the *product*. The product is said to be a *multiple* of both factors, and it is also *divisible* by both factors	Since $3 \times 23 = 69$, we can say that 3 and 23 are factors and 69 is the product, 69 is a multiple of both 3 and 23, and 69 is divisible by both 3 and 7.

Whenever an integer N is divisible by an integer x, we say that x is a *divisor* of N.

For the set of positive integers, any integer N that has exactly two distinct positive divisors, 1 and N, is said to be a *prime number*.

The first ten prime numbers are 2, 3, 5, 7, 11, 13, 17, 19, 23, and 29.

The integer 14 is **not** a prime number because it has four divisors: 1, 2, 7, and 14.

The integer 1 is **not** a prime number because it has only one positive divisor.

1.2.1 Fractions.

fraction is a number of the form $\frac{a}{b}$ where a and b are integers and $b \neq 0$. The a is called the *numerator* of the fraction, and b is called the *denominator*. Thus $\frac{9}{5}$ is a fraction having 9 as its numerator and 5 as its denominator. This technique can be used to add or subtract fractions. $\frac{a}{b}$ means $a \div b$. Thus b cannot be zero	
If the numerator and denominator of the fraction are both multiplied by the same integer, the resulting fraction will be equivalent to $\frac{a}{b}$	$\frac{7}{8} \times \frac{5}{5} = \frac{35}{40} = \frac{7}{8}$
To add or subtract two fractions with the same denominator, you simply add or subtract the numerators and keep the denominator the same.	$-\frac{7}{13} + \frac{6}{13} = \frac{-7+6}{13} = -\frac{1}{13}$ $\frac{7}{15} - \frac{6}{15} = \frac{7-6}{15} = \frac{1}{15}$

If the denominators are *not* the same, you may apply the technique mentioned above to make them the same before doing the addition or subtraction:	$\frac{4}{5}+\frac{3}{8}=\frac{4(8)+3(5)}{(5)(8)}=\frac{47}{40}$ $\frac{6}{9}+\frac{4}{3}=\frac{6+4(3)}{9}=\frac{18}{9}=2$ $\frac{10}{7}-\frac{5}{8}=\frac{10(8)-5(7)}{7x8}=\frac{80-35}{56}=\frac{35}{56}=\frac{5}{8}$
To multiply two fractions, multiply the two numerators and multiply the two denominators (the denominators need not be the same).	$\frac{5}{7}x\frac{4}{9}=\frac{(5)(4)}{(7)(9)}=\frac{20}{63}$
To divide one fraction by another, first *invert* the fraction you are dividing by, and then proceed as in multiplication.	$\frac{35}{42}\div\frac{15}{21}=\left(\frac{35}{42}\right)\left(\frac{21}{15}\right)=\frac{735}{630}=\frac{7}{6}=1\frac{1}{6}$
An expression such as $5\frac{2}{3}$ is called a **mixed fraction**	$5\frac{2}{3}$ means $5+\frac{2}{3}$ Therefore, $5\frac{2}{3}=5+\frac{2}{3}=\frac{15}{3}+\frac{2}{3}=\frac{17}{3}$

1.2.2 Decimals

Fractions with a power of ten as denominator are known as *Decimal fractions*. A decimal point is used and the place value for each digit corresponds to a power of 10. Decimals are written by omitting the denominator and inserting a decimal point in the numerator as many places on the right as there are ciphers of 10 in the denominator.	Example: the number 57.321 has five digits, where "5" is the "tens" digit; the place value for "5" is 10. "7" is the "units" digit; the place value for "7" is 1. "3" is the "tenths" digit; the place value for "3" is $\frac{1}{10}$ "2" is the "hundredths" digit; the place value for "2" is 1/100 "1" is the "thousandths" digit; the place value for "1" is1/1000 Therefore 57.321 is a short way of writing $(5)(10)+(7)(1)+(3)\left(\frac{1}{10}\right)+(2)\left(\frac{1}{100}\right)+(1)\left(\frac{1}{1000}\right)$
When adding or subtracting decimals, keep in mind to keep the decimal points under each other (line up the decimals)	324.6 + _67.4532_ 257.1468	536.7 - _65.657_ 471.043
When multiplying decimals, proceed as with whole numbers, then place the decimal point of the product as many places from the first number on the right as the sum of the decimal places in the multiplier and the multiplicand. It is not necessary to align the decimal points.	16.87 (2 decimal places) X _45.3_ (one decimal place) 6748 8435 5061 **764.211**(three decimal places)	13.46 (2 decimal places) X _22.45_ (2 decimal places) 6730 5384 2692 _**302.1770**_ (4 decimal places)

To divide a decimal by another, first move the decimal point in the divisor to the right to form a whole number. Then move the decimal point in the dividend the same number of places. This procedure determines the correct position of the decimal point in the dividend.	$184.4612 \div 16.324$ $\phantom{16324\sqrt{}}\underline{11.3}$ $16324\sqrt{184461.2}$ $\phantom{16324\sqrt{}}\underline{16324}$ $\phantom{16324\sqrt{1}}21221$ $\phantom{16324\sqrt{1}}\underline{16324}$ $\phantom{16324\sqrt{11}}48972$ $\phantom{16324\sqrt{11}}\underline{48972}$ $\phantom{16324\sqrt{111}}0$
To convert a common fraction to a decimal fraction, divide the numerator by the denominator and place the decimal point in the correct place	Since $\frac{a}{b}$ means $a \div b$ then fraction 5/9 means $5 \div 9$ $\underline{0.556}$ Thus $9\sqrt{5.0}$ $\underline{45}$ 50 $\underline{45}$ 50 $-\underline{45}$ 5 and so on
To convert a given decimal to an equivalent common fraction, place the entire number, as numerator, over the power of ten containing the same number of ciphers of 10 as there are decimal places. Cancel if possible to simplify.	1. $85.2 = \frac{852}{10}$ 2. $6.15 = \frac{615}{100}$ 3. $0.656 = \frac{656}{1000}$ This can further be simplified to $\frac{656 \div 8}{1000 \div 8} = \frac{82}{125}$

WARNING: *WRITING DECIMALS INCORRECTLY CAN LEAD TO MEDICATION ERRORS!! DO NOT WRITE TRAILLING ZEROS IF NOT NECESSARY. e.g. Write 5 and not 5.0 Write 0.5 and not .5 The latter is called a naked zero and the point may not be seen which can lead to 10-fold error!!*

1.2.3 Exponents

Exponents denote repeated multiplication of a number by itself. For example, 4^3 means 4x4x4 which equals 64. In the expression $4^3 = 64$, the number "3" is called the *exponent* of the *base* "4" and the expression is read as "four power three is sixty-four." The exponent tells us how many factors are in the product. When the exponent is 2, the number has been squared. Thus "$3^2 = 9$" is read "three squared" is nine.	$5^5 = (5)(5)(5)(5)(5)$ *or* $= 5 \times 5 \times 5 \times 5 \times 5$ $= 3125$ $-5^3 = (-5)\ (-5)\ (-5) = -125$ *Also* $(\frac{2}{3})^3 = (\frac{2}{3})(\frac{2}{3})(\frac{2}{3}) = \frac{8}{27}$

Exponents can be negative, zero or positive. Any number other than zero, with exponent zero equals 1. Thus $56^0= 1$. Any number other than zero with a negative exponent is equal to the reciprocal of the number	$m^0=1$ $\qquad$ $65^0=1$ $m^{-1}=\frac{1}{m}$ $\quad 43^{-2}=\frac{1}{43^2}$
The product of two or more powers of the same base is equal to that base with an exponent equal to the sum of the exponents of the powers	$m^y \times m^x = m^{y+x}$ $2^5 \times 2^4 = 2^{5+4} = 2^9$
The quotient of two powers of the same base is equal to that base with an exponent equal to the exponent of the dividend minus the exponent of the divisor	$\frac{m^x}{m^y} = m^{x-y}$ $3^8 \div 3^6 = 3^{8-6} = 3^2$ $5^2 \div 5^3 = 5^{2-3} = 5^{-1} = \frac{1}{5}$
The power of a power is found by multiplying the exponents	$(m^x)^y = m^{xy}$ $(2^2)^3 = 2^6 = 64$
The power of a product equals the product of the powers of the factors	$(2 \times 4 \times 3)^2 = 2^2 \times 4^2 \times 3^2 = 576$
The power of a fraction equals the power of the denominator	$= (\frac{2}{3})^2 = \frac{2^2}{3^2} = \frac{4}{9}$

1.2.4 Square roots

A *square root* of a positive number is a number which, when squared equals that number. For example, a square root of 16 is 4 because $4^2 = 16$. Another square root of 16 is −4 because $(-4)^2 = 16$. In fact, all positive numbers have two square roots that differ only in sign. The square root of 0 is 0 because $0^2 = 0$. Negative numbers do *not* have square roots because the square of a real number cannot be negative. If $N > 0$, then the positive square root of N is represented by $\sqrt{N}$, read "radical N." The negative square root of N, therefore, is represented by $-\sqrt{N}$.	**Rules of square roots:** If $a > 0$ and $b > 0$, then $(\sqrt{a})(\sqrt{b}) = \sqrt{ab}$ e.g. $(\sqrt{5})(\sqrt{6}) = \sqrt{5 \times 6} = \sqrt{30}$ e.g. $\frac{\sqrt{a}}{\sqrt{b}} = \sqrt{\frac{a}{b}}$ Example 1. $\frac{\sqrt{196}}{\sqrt{49}} = \sqrt{\frac{196}{49}} = \sqrt{4} = 2$ Example 2. $\frac{\sqrt{288}}{\sqrt{64}} = \sqrt{\frac{288}{64}} = \sqrt{\frac{12 \times 12 \times 2}{8 \times 8}} = \frac{12}{8}\sqrt{2}$ $= \frac{3}{2}\sqrt{2}$

The root of the power is found by dividing the exponent of the power by the index of the root	$\sqrt[3]{4^5} = 4^{\frac{5}{3}} =$
	$\sqrt[3]{8^9} = 8^{\frac{9}{3}} = 8^3 = 512$

1.2.5 Percent

In pharmacy calculations involving percentage are encountered very often. You may need to know the percent profit from sales, percent of the drug dose reaching the site of action, percent of production in the industry and so forth. You should therefore familiarize yourself with this principle.

The term Percent written as % means per hundred or divided by one hundred.

When we say 20 percent (20%) it means 20 parts in a total of 100 parts.

If you sell 30% of tablets from a tin of 1000 tablets, it means you have sold $\frac{30}{100}$ of 1000. Thus $\frac{30}{100} \times 1000 = 300$ tablets.

Percent is a ratio and therefore it has no units.

To change percent to a fraction the percent number becomes the numerator and 100 is the denominator	15% means $\frac{15}{100}$ Or 0.15 $300\% = \frac{300}{100}$ Or = 3 $0.05\% = \frac{0.05}{100} = 0.0005$
To Change a fraction to percent put the fraction in form of having 100 as its denominator, multiply by 100 so that the numerator becomes the percent	Change $\frac{1}{2}$ to percentage: $\frac{1}{2}\% = \frac{1}{2} \times 100 = 50\%$ Change $\frac{1}{8}$ to percentage: $\frac{1}{8}\% = \frac{1}{8} \times 100 = 2.5\%$ Convert 2.5 to percentage: $2.5 \times 100 = 250\%$ Express 0.9 as a percentage: $0.9 \times 100 = 90\%$
Q13. You may be asked to find out the value given the percentage. For example, What percent of 80 is 5?	This means you have 5 parts in 80 parts. Convert the total value to 100. Let the percent be x. then $\frac{5}{80} = \frac{x}{100}$ By cross multiplication, $80 \times X = 100 \times 5$ $80x = 500$ Therefore, $x = \frac{500}{80} = 6.25\%$ (Do not forget to put

	the % sign!!)
	Thus 5 is 6.25% of 80. The number 80 is called the base of the percent
	You may use a shortcut by dividing 5 to 80 and multiplying by 100 thus: $\frac{5}{80} x 100 = 6.25$
Q14. If the production of quinine tablets increased from 100,000 tablets per hour to 145.000 tablets per hour, what is the percent increase?	a. Find out the amount that has increased: $145,000 - 100,000 = 45,000$ b. Divide the amount to the original production and multiply by 100 $\frac{45,000}{100000} x\ 100 = 45\%$
Q15. The sale of erythromycin tablets fell from an average of five tins to 4 tins in the dry season, probably due to a decrease of infectious diseases. What was the percent decrease?	% decrease is found by dividing the amount of decrease $(5 - 4) = 1$ by the base ,5 or the larger and then multiply by 100: $\%\ Decrease = \frac{1}{4} x\ 100 = 20\%$ In other words, "4 is" 20% less than "5" In general, for any positive numbers x and y, where $x < y$ y is $(\frac{y-x}{y})(100)$ percent greater than x x is $(\frac{y-x}{x})(100)$ percent les than y • Note that in each of these statements, the base of the percent is in the denominator.
Q16. My monthly salary was increased by 8% to Shs 1,600.000/00 What was my salary before the increase?	$1600000 = 108\%$ What 100%? $\frac{1600000}{x} = \frac{108}{100}$ $X = 1,481,481$

1.2.6 Ratios and Proportions

Most calculations in pharmacy can be solved using **ratio and proportion**. Although to some people the concept of ratio and proportion appears to be intimidating, it is actually very simple when you break the process down into manageable steps

1.2.6.1 Ratio is a relative magnitude of two like quantities. We use ratios to make comparisons between two things. When we express ratios in words, we use the word "to" -- we say "the ratio of something to something else" --In layman's terms a ratio represents, simply, for every amount of one thing, how much there is of another thing. For example, suppose I have 10 pairs of socks for every pair of shoes then the ratio of shoes: socks would be 1:10 and the ratio of socks: shoes would be 10:1.

Ratios can be written in several different ways. The ratio of three kilograms to seven kilograms can be written:

    As a fraction e.g $\frac{3}{7}$

    Using the word "to" e.g "three to seven" (as used in the text above) or

    Using a colon e.g 3:7

Multiplying or dividing each term by the same nonzero number will give an equal ratio. For example, the ratio 2:4 is equal to the ratio 1:2. To tell if two ratios are equal, use a calculator and divide. If the division gives the same answer for both ratios, then they are equal. Thus

20:60 = 10:30 = 5:15 = 1:3

"30 to 20" is the same as "6 to 4" and also "3 to 2"

When two ratios have the same value, they are *equivalent*". For equivalent ratios, the product of the numerator of the one and the denominator of the other always equals the product of the denominator of the one and the numerator of the other	$\frac{20}{60} = \frac{1}{3}$ $20 \times 3 = 60 \times 1$
The numerator of one fraction is equal to the product of its denominator and the other fraction	If $\frac{5}{6} = \frac{15}{18}$ Then $5 = 6 \times \frac{15}{18}$ OR $\frac{6 \times 15}{18}$ Which is equal to 5
The denominator of the one equals the quotient of its numerator divided by the other fraction	Again if $\frac{5}{6} = \frac{15}{18}$ Then $6 = 5 \div \frac{15}{18}$ or $5 \times \frac{18}{15} = 6$

1.2.6.2 A Proportion is the expression of the equality of two proportions. A proportion simply states that two ratios are equal. We can write this in two different ways, the fraction form and the colon form. In the fraction form, the numerator and the denominator of one fraction have the same relationship as the numerator and denominator of another fraction. For example, 1/2 = 4/8; or, 1 is to 2 as 4 is to 8. The equal sign (=) is read as "as."

Using the colon form, the ratio to the left of the double colon is equal to the ratio to the right. As with the equal sign, the double colon is read as "as." For example, 1:2 :: 4:8; or 1 is to 2 as 4 is to 8.

Generally, proportions can be written as

1. a:b = c:d
2. a:b :: c:d
3. $\frac{a}{b} = \frac{c}{d}$

And read as *a is to b as c is to d*.

a and *d* are called *"extremes"* or outer numbers and *b* and *c* are the *"means"* or Middle members

1.2.7 CROSS MULTIPLICATION

In order to get two relationships, you have to cross-multiply.

If a = c as b = d, then ad = bc. How?

When you cross-multiply, you're really multiplying each side by n/n, where n is the denominator of the other side:

$$\frac{a}{b} = \frac{c}{d} \qquad \frac{a}{b} \times \left(\frac{d}{d}\right) = \frac{c}{d} \times \left(\frac{b}{b}\right)$$

Note that this doesn't change anything, because $\frac{d}{d} = 1$ and $\frac{b}{b} = 1$. Multiplying anything by 1 doesn't change its value. So now we have

$$\frac{ad}{bd} = \frac{bc}{bd} \qquad \text{Now both terms have the same denominator } bd$$

Since you're dividing both sides by the same thing, *bd*, you can ignore the denominator, to get

$$ad = bc$$

Once you get used to the idea, you can skip all the middle steps and just multiply the things that are crosswise from each other:

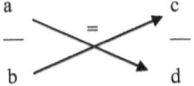 that is *ad = bc*

This is how we get the name **'cross-multiplying'**.

The product of the extremes is equal to the product of the means	If $\frac{a}{b} = \frac{c}{d}$ then $\quad ad = bc$
Therefore, among the four terms if one is unknown and the other three are known, it is easy to look for the missing term.	$a = \frac{bc}{d} \qquad b = \frac{ad}{c} \qquad c = \frac{ad}{b} \quad$ and $\quad d = \frac{bc}{a}$
Q17a. If 15 tablets of paracetamol have 7.5 grams of the active ingredient, how many tablets do we need to make a 100 mL syrup containing 10 gram of the active ingredient?	A tablet contains the active ingredient together with other substances called excipients that provide characteristics of that tablet. In this question we are asked to calculate a number of tablets

	containing 10 grams of paracetamol active ingredient. We are told that 15 tablets contain 7.5 grams of active ingredient paracetamol. We may arrange our problem as follows with same terms on one side $$\frac{15 \text{ tablets}}{y \text{ tablets}} = \frac{7.5 \text{ grams}}{10 \text{ grams}}$$ By cross multiplication, $y \times 7.5 = 15 \times 10$ $$y = \frac{15 \times 10}{7.5}$$ $$y = 20$$ Therefore, we need 20 tablets to make a 100 mL syrup containing 10 gram of paracetamol. This problem could also be solved by the following approach: $$y = 15 \div \frac{7.5}{10}$$ $$y = (15) \times \frac{10}{7.5}$$ $$y = 20$$
Q17b. Using the same analogy, if 15 tablets contain 7.5 gram of paracetamol, how many grams should be contained in 30 tablets?	$$= \frac{15 \text{ tablets}}{30 \text{ tablets}} = \frac{7.5 \text{ grams}}{y \text{ grams}} =$$ This is the same like saying $$\frac{(15 \text{ tablets})}{30 \text{ tablets}} \frac{\text{Contain } 7.5 \text{ grams}}{\text{contain } y \text{ grams}}$$ $$y = \frac{30 \times 7.5}{15}$$ $$y = 15$$
Q18. A 50 mg dose of a particular drug is prescribed. It is available in your pharmacy in 100 mg / 2 mL vials. What volume should be withdrawn from the vial to provide a 50 mg dose?	First, we need to determine exactly what the question is asking. In this case we want to know how many mL we need to provide a 50 mg dose of a particular drug. We know that we have 100 mg of

the drug (solute) in 2 mL (solution). The variable x in this case is the number of mL containing the 50 mg dose. Let's construct our ratio(s) and proportion:

100 mg : 2 mL : 50 mg : x mL

Multiply the means: 2 times 50 = 100
Multiply the extremes: 100 times x = 100x

$$2 \times 50 = 100x, \quad x = \frac{2 \times 50}{100} = 1$$

OR Divide both sides of the equation by the number before the x: $1 = x$

Therefore, we need to withdraw 1 mL to provide a 50 mg dose

Ratios should express relationship of denominate numbers of the same kind. In the above example, tablets are on one side and the number of grams is on the other side.

ALWAYS REMEMBER: SIMILAR UNITS ARE ON ONE SIDE:

e.g. $\frac{a \text{ (mL)}}{b \text{ (mL)}} = \frac{x \text{ (units)}}{y \text{ (units)}}$ NOT $\frac{a \text{ mL}}{y \text{ units}} = \frac{b \text{ mL}}{x \text{ units}}$

Most pharmaceutical calculations deal with simple ratios such as *Twice the cause, double the effect* or inversely such as *half the effect or half the concentration*.

Q19. 10 liters of a 10% w/v/ solution of ammonia were diluted to 20 liters with water. What is the percent strength the resulting dilution?	$\frac{10(liters)}{20(liters)} = \frac{x\%}{10\%}$ $$x = \frac{10 \times 10}{20}$$ $$x = 5\%$$ Percent strength of new dilution is 5% w/v

1.3 BASIC ALGEBRA

Algebra is about Translating words into algebraic expressions. This is a useful method of solving for an unknown quantity. The following are examples of how a problem can be translated into a mathematical expression in order to make it easy to solve.

Q19.

i.	A number increased by nine is fifteen	$x + 9 = 15$
ii.	Four less than a number is twenty	$x - 4 = 20$
iii.	Twice a number is eighteen	$2n = 18$
iv.	A number divided by 6 is eight	$\frac{k}{6} = 8$
v.	Twice a number, decreased by twenty-nine, is seven	$2t - 29 = 7$
vi.	Thirty-two is twice a number increased by eight	$32 = 2a + 8$
vii.	The quotient of fifty and five more than a number is ten	$\frac{50}{n+5} = 10$
viii.	Twelve is sixteen less than four times a number	$12 = 4x - 16$
ix. x.	Helen is x years old. In thirteen years she will be twenty-four years' old	$x + 13 = 24$
xi.	Each tablet of paracetamol costs 25 shillings. The price of h tablets of paracetamol is Two hundred fifty shillings.	$25h = 250$
xii.	Suzanne made a withdrawal of d shillings from her savings. Her old balance was Shs 350,000 and her new balance is Shs 280.	$350 - d = 280$
xiii.	A large pizza pie with 15 slices is shared among p students so that each student's share is 3 slices.	$\frac{15}{p} = 3$
xiv.	If the square of the number x is multiplied by 3, and then 10 is added to that product	$3x^2 + 10$
xv.	If your salary was to be increased by 20 percent what is your new salary	Let S be your present Salary. Your new salary is $s + \frac{20}{100}s = 1.2s$
xvi.	Suppose there are 15 students and p pairs of gloves. Distribute P pairs of gloves to 10 students so that each student gets 1 pair and the rest of the pairs of gloves are divided equally among the remaining 5 students. What will each of the 5 last students get?	$(\frac{p-10}{5})$
Q20. In the first semester you received the following scores in 3 pharmaceutics exams: 75, 74, and 45. What score will you need to attain on the next exam so that the average (arithmetic mean) for the 4 exams will be 75 which is "A")		If x represents the score on the next exam, then the arithmetic mean of 75 will be equal to $\frac{75 + 74 + 45 + x}{4} = 75$

	$$\frac{194 + x}{4} = 75$$ $$194 + x = 75 \times 4$$ $$x = (75 \times 4) - 194$$ X= 106%. *(which means it is impossible to attain this mark because it is more than 100%)*
Q21. An ointment containing 10 grams' calamine powder in Vaseline is 8% calamine. (by weight). How much Vaseline should be added to this ointment so that the ointment now has only 5% calamine?	*If 10 gram of calamine powder = 8% or 8/100 of the total weight of ointment, Vaseline should be 92%.* *By proportion* $\frac{10}{x} = \frac{8}{92}$ *where x is the weight of Vaseline.* *Solving for x, $8x = 92 \times 10 = 920$. $x = 115g$* *Let y represent the number of grams of Vaseline to be added. Therefore, the total number of grams of Vaseline in the new ointment will be $115 + y$ and the total number of grams of new ointment will be $115 + y + 10$ in total. Since the new mixture must be 5% calamine* $$\frac{10}{(115+y+10)} \times 100 = 5$$ $$\frac{10 \times 100}{115 + y + 10} = 5$$ *Therefore $1000 = 5(115+y+10)$* $$1000 = 5(125 + y)$$ $$= 625 + 5y$$ $$5y = 1000 - 625$$ $$y = 375$$ *Therefore, add 375 gram of Vaseline to obtain 5% ointment.*
Q22. If it takes 3 hours for machine A to produce N tablets of metronidazole, and it takes machine B only 2 hours to do the same job, how long would it take to do the job if both machines worked simultaneously?	*Since machine A takes 3 hours to do the job, machine A can do $\frac{1}{3}$ of the job in 1 hour.* *Similarly, machine B can do $\frac{1}{2}$ of the job in 1 hour.* *And if we let x represent the number of hours it would take for the machines working simultaneously to do the job, the two machines would do $\frac{1}{x}$ of the job in 1 hour. Therefore,*

	$\frac{1}{3}+\frac{1}{2}=\frac{1}{x}$ $\quad$ $\frac{1(2)}{2x3}+\frac{1(3)}{2x3}=\frac{5}{6}=\frac{1}{x}$ $x=\frac{6}{5}=1\frac{1}{5}$ hours [We know that $\frac{1}{5}$ hrs = 12 min] It will take both machines 1 hour and 12 minutes to do the job when working simultaneously.
Q23. It costs One Pharmaceutical Company 120 shillings to produce each of Erythromycin tablet, and it is assumed that if 10,000 tablets were produced, all will be sold. What must be the selling price per tablet to ensure that the *profit* (revenue from sales minus total cost to produce) on the 10,000 tablets is greater than Tshs 800,000	If y represents the selling price per tablet, then the profit per tablet is y-120. The total profit for 1000 tablets is 10,000 (y – 120). In order to realize more profit than this amount the selling price must be in such a way that 10,000(y-120) > 800,000 Solving the equation, $\quad$ y-120 > 800,000 /10,000 $\quad$ y- 120 > 80 $\quad\quad$ y > 80 – -120) $\quad\quad$ y > 200 The selling price must therefore be greater than 200 TShs
Q24. Find an algebraic expression to represent each of the following. $\quad$ (a) The square of y is subtracted from 5, and the result is multiplied by 37.	$37(5-y^2) = 185 - y$
$\quad$ (b) Three times x is squared, and the result is divided by 7.	$\frac{(3x)^2}{7} = \frac{9x}{7}$
$\quad$ (c) The product of $(x + 4)$ and y is added to 18.	$18 + (x+4)y = 18 + xy + 4y$
Q25. For a given two-digit positive integer, the tens digit is 5 greater than the units digit. The sum of the digits is 13. Find the integer.	Let the tens digit be x and let the units digit be y $\quad$ (i) $\quad$ x= y+5 $\quad$ (ii) $\quad$ x+y =13 Taking the value of x from (i), $\quad$ y+5+y=13 $\quad$ 2y +5 = 13. Thus $y = \frac{13-5}{2} = \frac{8}{2} = 4$ But from (i), x = y+5 $\quad\quad$ x = 4+5 = 9 if x =9 and y = 4, The integer therefore is 94
Q26. If the ratio of 2x to 5y is 3 to 4, what is the ratio of x to y?	2x:5y = 3:4

	$$\frac{2x}{5y} = \frac{3}{4}$$ $\frac{x}{y} = \frac{3 \times 5}{4 \times 2} = \frac{15}{8}$ *Thus the ratio x:y = 15:8* *You can prove by substituting x and y in the original equation, 2x:5y = 3:4* *(2x15) :(5x8) = 30:40 = 3:4*
Q27. Mucolyn syrup pediatric is sold at half the adult formula Mucolyn. If 5 adult bottles and 8 children's bottles cost a total of Tshs 27,000, what is the cost of an adult Bottle?	Let the children bottle price be x. Then the Adult bottle price will be 2x *(2x) (5) + 8x = 27,000.* *10x + 8x = 27,000* *18x = 27,000 x= 1500* Children bottle cost 1500 Shillings and adult bottle cost 3000 Shillings.
Q 28. I have banked a total of 3 million shillings. Part of the money is in a fixed deposit in Bank A and yields 10% interest per year, and the rest is in bank B yielding 8% interest per year. If the total yearly interest from this investment is 256,000 shillings, how much did I invest at 10% and how much at 8%?	Let the money in bank A be x and the money in Bank B be y. *x+y = 3,000,000* *The interest from money* $x = \frac{10}{100}x = 0.1x$ *The interest on money y* $=\frac{8}{100}x = 0.08y$ *0.1x + 0.08y = 256,000* (total interest) Combining the two equations we get: 1) x + y = 3,000.000 2) 0.1x + 0.08y = 256,000 Multiply equation 1 by 10, and equation 2 by 100, and subtract equation 2 from equation 1: 1) 10x + 10y = 30,000,000 2) <u>10x + 8y = 25,600,000</u> 2y = 4,400,000 *y= 2,200,000 shillings (money invested at 8% interest)* if x +y = 3,000.000, then x = 3,000,000- 2,200,000 **x = 800,000 shillings (money invested at 10% interest)**

CHAPTER 2

Interpretation of Prescriptions

The term Prescription is defined as "an order for medication issued by a medical practitioner (Doctor of medicine, dental surgeon, veterinarian or other properly licensed medical practitioners)" which designate medications and dosage to be prepared or dispensed by a pharmacist and administered to a particular patient. Medications thus dispensed are also referred to as Prescriptions.

A prescription may have one or more medicines ordered. The medicines may be ready made (also known as prefabricated) such as tablets, capsules or syrups from a pharmaceutical company, or a dispenser may be required to compound or admixture ingredients to make a medicine in a required concentration and quantity.

2.1 Features of a prescription:

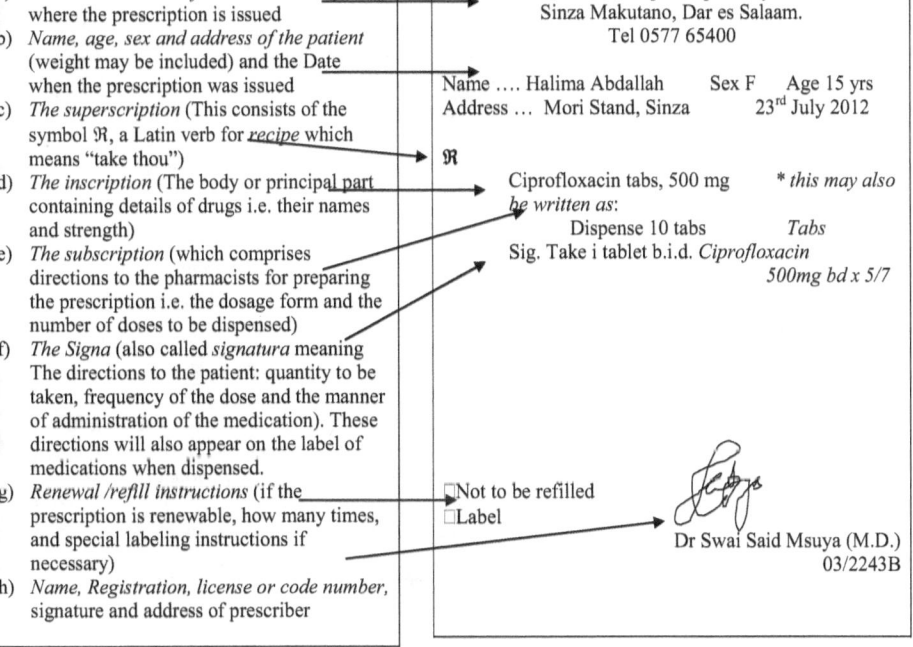

a) *Name and address of the clinic* or hospital where the prescription is issued
b) *Name, age, sex and address of the patient* (weight may be included) and the Date when the prescription was issued
c) *The superscription* (This consists of the symbol ℞, a Latin verb for *recipe* which means "take thou")
d) *The inscription* (The body or principal part containing details of drugs i.e. their names and strength)
e) *The subscription* (which comprises directions to the pharmacists for preparing the prescription i.e. the dosage form and the number of doses to be dispensed)
f) *The Signa* (also called *signatura* meaning The directions to the patient: quantity to be taken, frequency of the dose and the manner of administration of the medication). These directions will also appear on the label of medications when dispensed.
g) *Renewal /refill instructions* (if the prescription is renewable, how many times, and special labeling instructions if necessary)
h) *Name, Registration, license or code number,* signature and address of prescriber

Fig 1. Features of a prescription

Prescriptions are usually written on a pre-printed form containing the following information:

2.1.2 Information on Prescription:

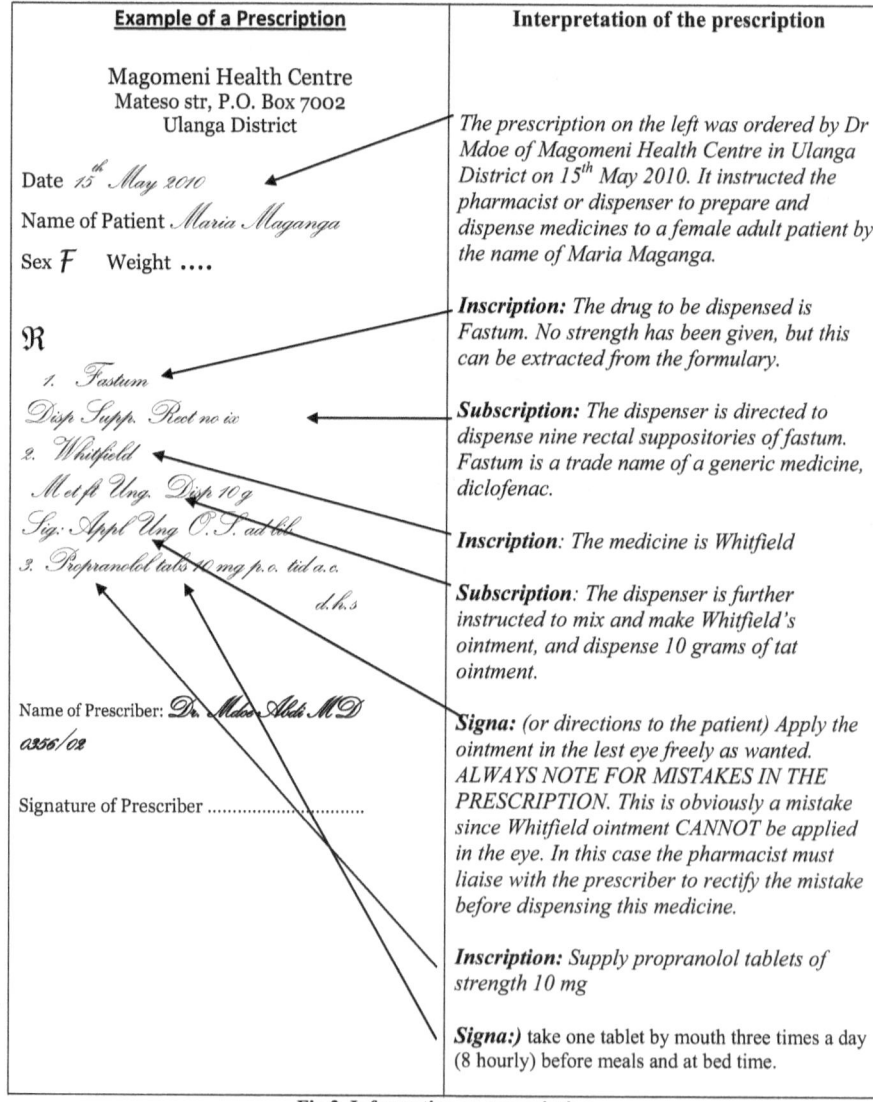

Fig 2. Information on prescription

2.2 COMMON LATIN ABBREVIATIONS AND THEIR MEANING

Abbreviation	Meaning	Latin
aa	of each	ana
a.c.	before meals	ante cibum
a.	right ear	aurio dextra
ad.lib.	freely as wanted	ad libitum
admov	apply	admove
agit	stir/shake	agita
alt. h.	every other hour	alternis horis
a.m.	morning, before noon	ante meridian
amp.	Ampoule	
amt	Amount	
aq.	water	aqua
a.l., a.s	Left ear aurio laeva,	aurio sinister
b.i.d.	twice a day	bis in die
B.M.	Bowel movement	
Bolus	Very large single dose	
cap.	capsule	capsula
c with bar on top	with	cum
c	food	cibos
cc	with food	cum cibos
comp.	compound	
crm , cr	cream	
D5W	Dextrose 5% solution	
DNS	Dextrose in normal saline	
Dc, D/C, disc	Discontinue	
Dil.	Dilute	
Disp.	Dispense	
div.	divide	divide
D.W.	Distilled water	
e.m.p	as directed	ex modo prescripto
eq.pts.	equal parts	equalis partis
ft	make, let it be made fiat	
g	gram	
gtt.	a drop	gutta
h.	hour	hora
h.s.	bed time	hora somni
IM	intra muscular injection	
Inj	Injection	
IV	Intravenous	
Lin	Liniment	
Lot	Lotion	
mcg	Microgram	
mEq	Milliequivalent	
mg	Milligram	
Mist	Mixture	Mistura
Nebul.	Spray	nebula
no.	number	numero
noct.	At night	noctura
NS	Normal saline	
O	pint	octarius
o.d.	right eye	oculus dexter
o.s	left eye	oculus sinister
o.u.or O_2	both eyes	oculus uterque
p.m.	evening or afternoon	post meridien

p.r.n.	as omLasion requires	pro re nata
p.o.	orally	per os
p.r	by rectum	
q.s.	a sufficient quantity	quantum sufficiat
q4h	every 4 hours	quaque 4 hora
q6h	every 6 hours	quaque 6 hora
qld	every day	quaque 1 die
qlw	every week	
q.h.s.	every night at bedtime	quaque hora somni
q.i.d.	four times a day	quater in die
RL	Ringer Lactate solution	
s.i.d.	once a day	semel in die
Sig., S.	write on the label	signa
SOB	Shortness of breath	
stat.	immediately	statim
supp	suppository	
tab.	a tablet	tabella
t.i.d.	three times a day	ter in die
tsp	teaspoon	
tr	Tincture	
tbsp	table spoon	
top.	Topical	
TPN	Total parenteral Nutrition	
Ung.	Ointment	Unguentum
USP	United States Pharmacopoeia	
UTI	Urinary tract infection	
w/o	Without	

2.2.1 Examples of Subscriptions (Directions to the pharmacists)

Q30. Interprete the following subscriptions:

Ft. supp.no xv	= Make 15 suppositories
M. ft. cap d.t.d no xviii	= Mix and make capsules. Give 18 such doses.
M et ft pulv. Div in dos. # C	= Mix and make powder. Divide into 100 doses.
M. et div. in pulv no xxxv	= Mix and divide into 35 powders.
M. isoton.sol. Disp ℥ii	= Make an isotonic solution and dispense 12 fluidounces.
Disp. tal. dos. xii. N.R.	= Dispense such twelve doses. Do not repeat
M. et ft. inj. For I.V. use.	= Mix and make an injection for intravenous use.
M. et ft sol. DTD Lv	= Mix and make a solution and give such 55 doses
M. et ft mist. 1g/tbsp	= Mix and make a mixture containing one gram per tablespoon.
Ft. cap.# 1. Disp. tal. no xxiv non rep.	= make a capsule. Dispense 24 such doses. Do not repeat.
Disp .sup. rect. no. vi	= Dispense six rectal Suppositories
Label GTN 300mcg	= Label Glyceryl Trinitrate 300 microgram

2.2.2 Examples of Signas (directions to the patient)

Q31. Interprete the following signas:

Tab ii q 6h ATC UTI = Take two tablets around the clock for treatment of urinary tract infection.
tsp ii ex aq. q.4-6 h p.r.n. nausea = take two tablets in water every four to six hourly to treat nausea.
Caps ii q.i.d. p.c. et h.s. = Take two capsules four (4) times a day after each meal and at bedtime.

gtt ii o.d. q.d. a.m. 5/7	= Instill two drops in the right eye every day in the morning for five days.
gtt ii o.u. q.6 h p.r.n. pain.	= instill two drops in each eye every six hours as needed to treat pain
Tab i sublingually, rep p.r.n.	= place one tablet sublingually and repeat as necessary.
Apply noct. for pain e.m.p.	= apply at night for pain as directed
inhale nebul p.r.n SOB	= inhale the spray as necessary for shortness of breath.
Appl. ung. O_2 ad.lib	= Apply the ointment in both eyes as much as you desire.

Further examples of interpretations of prescriptions:

Q32. *Interprete the following prescriptions:*

Phenobarbitone 30 mg p.o. q.d h.s. rep s.o.s = Take phenobarbitone 30 mg orally everyday at bedtime. Repeat if there is a need.

Metakelfin ii tabs stat. Rpt after 1/52 = Take 2 metakelfin tablets at once. Repeat the dose after 1 week.

Amoxycillin caps 1 gm stat; 500 mg tds x 7d a.c = Take four capsules of amoxicillin (containing 250 mg each) immediately, then take two capsules eight hourly (three times a day) before meals daily for the next seven days.

1L DNS I.V. c Vit B_{12} = Infuse 1 liter of Dextrose saline with vitamin B_{12} intravenously.

Azithromycin suspension 7.5 mL bd p.c. 5/7 = Azithromycin suspension 7.5 mL (1 ½ teaspoon) every 12 hours (twice daily) for five days.

1 L ORS ad.lib. disc after 24 hr = Reconstitute 1 liter of oral rehydration salts. Take liberally and discard the remaining contents after 24 hours.

Laprazolam tabs 1 mg 1 tab h.s. p.r.n. sleep = Administer laprazolam tablets of 1 mg each before bed time when required for sleep.

Motilium susp. 5 mL t.i.d 2/7 N&V = Take 5 mL of motilium suspension eight hourly (three times a day) for Nausea and vomiting.

D5W + 20 mEq KCl at 84 mL /hr = Administer 20 mEq of potassium chloride per liter in dextrose 5% in water at the rate of 84 mL per hour.

Vincristine SO_4 1mg/m^2 BSA = Dispense Vincristine sulphate at the dose of 1 mg per square meter of the body surface area.

2.3 Roman Numerals

The use of Roman numerals dates back to ancient times when symbols were used for pharmaceutical computations and record keeping. Some physicians still use Roman numerals in dosage calculations; therefore, in order to read and fill prescriptions correctly, pharmacy dispensers must understand Roman numerals.

The Romans depicted numbers using eight letters of the alphabet as follows:

(a) ss = ½   *Numbers below fifty Can appear in low or upper case

(b) I or i = 1   (c) V or v = 5   (d) X or x = 10   (e) L = 50   (f) C = 100   (g) D = 500   (h) M = 1000

The most common letters you will use are those between 1/2 (ss) and 10 (x). The letters L, C, D, and M are rarely used in practice, and are shown above for your review.

ss = ½
(i) = 1   (ii) = 2   (iii) = 3   (iv) = 4   (v) = 5
(vi) = 6   (vii) = 7   (viii) = 8   (ix) = 9   (x) = 10   xv = 15   xx = 20   xxx = 30

How to form Numbers

At their simplest, numbers are formed by stringing the letters together to add up to the number required. Like this: ii = 2   xxx = 30   xii = 12   CXXIII = 123

The rule is to use the biggest numeral possible at each stage, so 15 is represented by xv not vvv nor xiiiii. It follows from this rule that numerals always go from left to right in descending order. This could still lead to some very long strings. For example, using this rule 99 would be LXXXXVIIII. So a new rule was invented. A smaller value letter to the left of a larger value one is subtracted. So 4 becomes iv - which is 5 minus 1 - rather than iiii. Roman numerals of the same value can be repeated in sequence, only up to three times. When you can no longer repeat, you need to subtract.

There are three rules about these smaller numerals which are placed to the left of a bigger one and subtracted:

1. The subtractive numeral to the left must be I, X, or C. The 'five' numerals V, L, and D cannot be used or repeated in sequence because when their values are doubled, they become separate Roman numerals). M cannot be used because it is the biggest numeral anyway.

2. The subtracted number must be no less than a tenth of the value of the number from which it is subtracted. So an X can be placed to the left of a C or an L but not to the left of an M or a D. The correct way of looking at this rule is that each power of ten is dealt with separately. So 49 is XLIX, not IL.

3. Normally, only one smaller number can be placed to the left. So 19 can be depicted XIX but 17 cannot be written XIIIX or IIIXX.

CHAPTER 3

Weights and Measures

3.1 Introduction.

In pharmacy courses, be it a certificate, diploma or a degree course, and indeed in the practice of pharmacy, we must be able to prepare medicines, a process known as **Extemporaneous preparation**. The term **Compounding** is also used synonymously to express preparation of extemporaneous medicines. We prepare medicines in form of liquids such as solutions, mixtures, lotions, syrups and emulsions. We may also be asked to prepare a liquid preparation given solid medicines. For this purpose, a pharmacy student or practitioner needs to be very conversant with systems of measures and weights so as to prepare medicines accurately and appropriately. Therefore, students must learn manipulation of **balances** and **weights**, as well as appropriately use **measures** (graduated flasks and pippets). We expect that actual manipulations and skills are dealt with in practical classes. This manual deals with the calculation part.

In the past, each country had its system of measurement and weight for the purpose of trade. But worldwide there were two **Common systems**, namely the Avoirdupois and Apothecary systems as adopted from the UK and the USA. The avoirdupois system was used in everyday life, whereas, as the name suggests, the apothecary system, was used by pharmacists and alchemists. The main usage of the Apothecary system was measurement of VOLUMES (while Avoirdupois systems was applied in WEIGHTS)

Both Avoirdupois and the Apothecary systems have now been replaced, for the most part, by the **metric system**. The reason of change was necessitated by the fact that the Avoirdupois and Apothecary systems have units which are not interrelated and used to bring confusion. In the 18th century many countries began pondering about harmonizing and standardizing Units of weights and measures. The French metric system seemed to be the choice. The Metric system was advantageous because it was logical. It consists of a standard set of inter-related base units and a standard set of prefixes in powers of ten. These base units are used to derive larger and smaller units and replaced a huge number of unstandardized units of measure that existed in the avoirdupois and apothecary systems. In the metric system the table of length, volume and weight are conveniently correlated, because the meter is the fundamental unit of the system.

The Metric system was legalized in Great Britain in 1864 and two years later, United States followed suit. In 1960 the metric system was recognized by the World as the International System of units (referred to SI units) to be used by all countries. All countries adopted the Units. But some habits are hard to die. Although SI units are official worldwide, to date UK, USA and some other countries still use the old systems in daily use. In the UK for instance, beer is sold in pints, the area of land is still in acres and the distance is measured in miles. Some physicians prefer to use Latin inscriptions and some old units in writing their prescriptions. Thus some prescriptions may have the weights or volumes expressed in units of one of the common systems. Therefore, students must still learn the old units. It is for this reason that we are compelled to continue teaching the old systems the so called **Common systems** so that should you come across such units you can still apply your professional knowledge in preparing medicines.

3.2 METRIC SYSTEM

The **metric system** is an international decimalized system of measurement of volumes, weights and length based on Liters, Grams and Meters as fundamental units. The metric system is a simple, adaptable and brief system that allows easy conversion. Among the merits of the system are:
1. Every weight and measure bears a simple relation to the initial unit. Thus the tables of metric conversions are simple, based on decimal system of notation, and the greater of two consecutive denominations of the same kind is always ten times less.
2. Every unit is a multiplied or divided by the same number, (i.e. 10) to obtain the various denominations and the increase or decrease is expressed by simply moving a decimal point.
3. Units of weight, length and volume are commensurable e.g. 10 mL of water weigh 10 grams, 30 mL weigh 30 grams and 1 liter of water (1000 mL) weigh 1 kilogram (1000 grams).
4. It is a universally or internationally accepted system which is used Worldwide

Each table of the metric system contains a definitive unit. The *meter* is the unit of length, the *liter* of volume and the *gram* of weight. The prefixes which indicate multiplication are of Greek derivation (deca, hector, kilo, mega, giga, tera, peta and exam). The divisions of the units are expressed by Latin prefixes (deca, cent, mille, micro, nana, picot, feta and atom)

Table 1. Metric intercorversions

Prefixes		WEIGHT		Linear measure (Unit = meter, m)		Liquid measure	
		(unit = Gram, g)				(unit = Liter, L)	
Attu-	= 1 quintillionth = 10^{-18}	attogram	ag	attometer	Am	attoliter	Al
Femto-	= 1 quadrillionth = 10^{-15}	femtogram	fg	femtometer	Fm	femtoliter	Fl
Pico-	= 1 trillionth = 10^{-12}	picogram	pg	picometer	Pm	picoliter	Pl
Nano-	= 1 billionth = 10^{-9}	nanogram	ng	nanometer	Nm	nanoliter	Nl
Micro-	= 1 millionth = 10^{-6}	microgram	μg or mcg	micrometer	μm	microliter	μL
Milli-	= 1 thousandth = 10^{-3}	milligram	mg	millimeter	mm	milliliter	ML
Centi-	= 1 hundredth = 10^{-2}	centigram	cg	centimeter	Cm	centiliter	Cl
Deci-	= 1 tenth = 10^{-1}	decigram	dg	decimeter	Dm	deciliter	Dl
		gram	g	meter	M	Liter	L
Deka-	= x ten = x10	decagram	Dg	decameter	Dm	decaliter	DL
Hecto-	= x one hundred = 10^{2}	hectogram	hg	hectometer	Hm	hectoliter	Hl
Kilo-	= x one thousand = $x10^{3}$	kilogram	kg	kilometer	Km	kiloliter	Kl
Myria-	= x ten thousand = x 10^{4}	myriagram	myg	myriameter	mym	myrialiter	myL
Mega-	= x one million = x 10^{6}	megagram	Mg	megameter	Mm	megaliter	ML
Giga-	= x one billion = x 10^{9}	gigagram	Gg	gigameter	Gm	gigaliter	GL
Tera	= x trillion = x 10^{12}	teragram	Tg	terameter	Tm	teraliter	TL
Peta-	= x quadrillion = x 10^{15}	petagram	Pg	petameta	Pm	petalita	PL
Exa-	= x quintillion = 10^{18}	exagram	Eg	exameter	Em	Exaliter	EL

WEIGHT	LENGTH	VOLUME
1 gram = 0.001 kilogram	1 meter = 0.001 km	1 liter = 0.001 kiloliter
= 0.01 hektogram	= 0.01 hektometer	= 0.01 hektoliter
= 0.1 dekagram	= 0.1 dekameter	= 0.1 dekaliter
= 10 decigrams	= 10 decimeters	= 10 deciliters
= 100 centigrams	= 100 centimeters	= 100 centiliters
= 1000 m illigram	= 1000 m illimeters	= 1000 m illiliters
= 1,000,000 micrograms	= 1,000,000 micrometers	= 1,000,000 microliters
= 1,000,000,000 nanogram	= 1,000,000,000 nanometers	= 1,000,000,000 nanoliters

For weights, the denominations most commonly used are the microgram, milligram, gram and kilogram. When measuring length, the most commonly used denominations are millimeter, centimeter and meter. Lastly, for volumes the most commonly used denominations are milliliter and liter.

Table 2 Common Metric units

Common Weight conversions	Common Length Conversion	Common Volume conversion
1000 μg or mcg = 1 milligram	1000 mm = 100 cm	1000 ML = 1 L
1000 mg = 1 gram	100 cm = 1 m	
1000g = 1 Kg		

Q33. I have banked a total of shillings 3 million. Part of the money is in a fixed deposit in Bank A and yields 10 percent interest per year, and the rest is in a savings account in Bank B yielding 8 percent interest per year. If the total yearly interest from this investment is Shillings 256,000 how much did I invest at 10 percent and how much at 8 percent?	Let the money in bank A be x, and the money in Bank B be y $x + y = 3$ million The interest from money $x = x\frac{10}{100} = 0.1x$ The interest from Money $y = y\frac{8}{100} = 0.8y$ $0.1x + 0.08Y = 256,000$ Multiply by 100 on both sides, (1) $10X + 8y = 25,600,000$ Also recall $x + y = 3000000$. Multiply by 10 on both sides, (1) $\underline{10X + 10y = 30000000}$ Subtract equation (2) from (1) $2y = 4,400,000$. **Y = 2,200,000** But $x + y = 3,000,000$ therefore, $x = 3000000 - 2200000$ **X = 800,000 shillings**.

3.3 USING BALANCES.

3.3.1 Determination of Minimum weighable quantity on balances

Determination of potential errors and minimum weighable quantity given acceptable committable error

In compounding it is very important to ensure accuracy in weights and measures. Mistakes in measuring or weighing are never acceptable in pharmacy. Accuracy may be lost particularly if you are dealing with very small quantities, such as those found with very potent medicines, toxic medicines and adjuvants needed in minute quantities, such as dyes and flavors.

When using prescription balances, you should know its sensitivity and therefore be able to determine the smallest weighable quantity and estimating the percentage error in weighing.

Measurements are never 100% accurate. When you use a balance and weigh 50 milligrams it could be +/_ a certain amount albeit small but not negligible. Therefore, a pharmacist must be able to know the magnitude of errors made during weighing and measuring. This will depend on the **sensitivity** of the balance that you are using. The excess or deficiency from the actual weight is the "potential error". Thus if you use a torsion balance, whose "sensitivity" is 5 mg, the actual weight is 50 mg +/_ 5 mg, i.e. the actual weight may be 45 mg or 55 mg. The **maximum potential error** is +/_ 5 or simply 5.

The percentage error is the maximum potential error multiplied by 100 and divided by the desired quantity:

$$\text{Percentage error} = \frac{(error) \times 100\%}{Desired\ Quantity}$$

In the above example, whereby the maximum potential error is 5, if we want to weigh 50 mg, the percentage error shall be $\frac{5 \times 100}{50}$ = 10%. Such a percentage error is unacceptable in pharmacy. 5% error is acceptable

Note that the word *sensitivity* may be used to mean the smallest possible weight that that will disturb the balance. *Sensitivity requirement* is defined as the maximum change in load that will cause a specified change one subdivision on the index plate from the state of rest. The latter designates the sensitiveness of the balance.

If the balance that you are using is suspiciously inaccurate, you may countercheck it with a balance of a higher accuracy, and from the difference in weight between the two balances, approximate potential error may be measured.

Suppose you use a balance in your pharmacy to weigh 900 mg of a substance. Later on you countercheck the weight by using a more sensitive balance from Chemistry department, and you find that the weight is actually 850mg. This means in the first weighing there was an excess of 50 mg. You may calculate percentage error as follows:

$$\text{Percentage error} = \frac{(error) \times 100\%}{Desired\ Quantity}$$

$$= \frac{50}{900} \times 100 = 5.56\%$$

You may also be asked to calculate the smallest quantity that can be measured within a desired accuracy. Suppose you have a balance which is sensitive to 8 mg and you are asked to calculate the smallest quantity that can be weighed on this balance with a potential error of not more than 6%. You may proceed using the following formula:

$$\textbf{Smallest quantity weighable on a balance} = \frac{\textbf{100 x Maximum potential error}}{\textbf{Permissible percentage error}}$$

$$= \frac{100 \times 8\ mg}{6} = 133.33 mg$$

The balance sensitivity is also a point where you can commit the maximum error in weighing.

Q34. Calculate the percent maximum potential error that you will encounter if you attempt to weigh 150 mg on a balance with sensitivity requirement of 5 mg	$\text{Percentage error} = \frac{(\text{error}) \times 100\%}{\text{Desired Quantity}}$ $= \frac{5 \times 100}{150} = 3.3\%$ Answer
Q35. The sensitivity requirement of a balance is 0.006 g. what will be the percentage error if you use this balance to weigh o,1 g	$\frac{0.006 \times 100}{0.1} = 6\%$ Answer.
Q36. A student weighed atropine sulphate on one balance and obtained 0.375 g. His teacher later gave him a more accurate balance which he used and obtained 0.400 g. Calculate the percent error he made with the first balance	The weight used to calculate the percentage error is the weight obtained by the balance whose error is sought for, i.e. 0.375 mg and not 0.400 mg $\frac{0.025}{0.375} \times 100 = 6.67\%$ Answer
Q37. A student attempted to decant 60 mL of glycerin from a measuring cylinder containing 100 mL of glycerin. Later he noted that actually what was left in the measuring cylinder was 45 mL. Calculate the percentage error he made.	The error was 5 mL $\text{Percentage error} = \frac{(\text{error}) \times 100\%}{\text{Desired Quantity}}$ $= \frac{5 \times 100}{60} = 8.3\%$ Answer.
Q38. A Prescription balance has a sensitivity requirement of 4 mg. What the smallest amount that can be weighed on this balance with a potential error of not more than 2.5%?	$\text{Smallest quantity weighable on a balance} = \frac{100 \times \text{Maximum potential error}}{\text{Permissible percentage error}}$ $\frac{100 \times 4}{2.5} = 160\ mg$ Answer.
Q39. The sensitivity requirement of a balance is 15 mg. What is the smallest amount weighable with a potential error of not more than 2 %?	$\text{Smallest quantity weighable on a balance} = \frac{100 \times \text{Maximum potential error}}{\text{Permissible percentage error}}$ $\frac{100 \times 15}{2} = 750\ mg$ or $0.75g$. Answer.

3.4 Measuring minute quantities: Aliquot Method

The aliquot method of weighing is used to weigh small quantities of substances, within the degree of accuracy desired, especially very potent substances which are required in minute quantities. Such substance could be weighed using expensive precision balances, which are normally not found in pharmacies. Normal prescription balances may not be sensitive enough to measure such minute quantities accurately and precisely, and a bigger error will be committed. Such potent substances include coloring agents, volatile oils, and potent drugs such as chlorpheniramine, morphine and atropine sulphate.

An aliquot part is a part that is contained in a whole number of times in a quantity. For example, if you have 2mg of atropine in 10mg of lactose and atropine, the amount of atropine is the fifth aliquot ($\frac{10}{2} = 5$)

Any number of parts may be chosen but frequently and for convenience sake a multiple of 10 is used. Factors used to choose the multiple include sensitivity of the used balance, convenience of multiplying, availability of weights and the cost of the substance to be measured.

3.4.1 How to weigh using aliquot method:

Practical Problem: The balance available in your pharmacy has a sensitivity requirement of 5 mg. Supply Atropine Sulphate in 5 mg doses with an accuracy of 5% (+/_)

Prescription balances are not sensitive enough to weigh 5 mg accurately. Therefore, do not attempt to use such a balance for this purpose.

Step 1: Determine the minimum weighable quantity of your balance in order to measure the quantity of the substance that can be weighed with the available balance. In this case, the balance sensitivity = 5, and permissible percent error = 5%,

$$Smallest\ quantity\ weighable = \frac{100 \times Maximum\ potential\ error}{Permissible\ percentage\ error}$$

$$= \frac{100 \times 5}{5} = 100mg$$

Thus the minimum weighable quantity for this balance is 100 mg.

Step 2: Determine how much of the active ingredient you are going to weigh. This amount should be equal to or more than the minimum weighable quantity for it to be weighed accurately. Ask yourself how many aliquots do you want to make? Suppose you want to make a powder that will be divided in 10 parts to provide 5 mg of atropine (i.e. you want to make a 10th Aliquot), then amount of atropine needed = 5x 10 =50 mg. This is not an accurately weighable amount as it is less than the minimum weighable quantity. Let us make the aliquot part to be 20th i.e. the final powder shall be divided into 20 parts so as to provide 5 mg in each part. Then the amount of atropine required is

20 x 5= 100 mg.

This is a weighable amount (100 mg is the minimum weighable amount)

Step 3: Choose the amount of the pack that will contain the amount of the active ingredient required. In this example we require each dose to have 5 mg atropine. Calculate the quantity of the inert substance required to dilute the active component, so that on dividing, each part shall contain the desired amount of atropine in each dose, i.e. 5 mg

Suppose we choose that our pack shall weigh 120 mg (which is above the minimum weighable quantity). This 120 mg shall contain 5 mg Atropine, and the rest (120-5=115) shall be the inert substance.

Amount of Atropine sulphate = 5 mg x 20packs	= 100 mg
Amount of inert substance (lactose) = 115 mg x 20 packs	= 2300 mg
Total =	= 2400 mg

Step 4: Weigh the active ingredient (100 mg atropine) and the inert substance (2300 mg lactose) and mix them thoroughly.

Step 5: Weigh 120 mg of the mixed powder and pack. Each of the pack shall have 115 mg lactose and 5 mg atropine.

NOTE THAT THE CHOSEN AMOUNTS ARE CONVENIENTLY WEIGHABLE.

In the above example if we chose the final pack to weigh 150 mg, for 20 packs the calculation would be as follows:

1. Atropine shall still be 5 mg x 20 packs = 100 mg

2. Inert substance (lactose) shall be (wt. of the pack – wt. of active ingredient) = 150 mg – 5 mg =145 mg

   Total quantity of inert substance for 20 packs = 145mg x20 = 2900 mg

3. Weigh 100 mg of active ingredient and 2900 mg of inert substance and mix thoroughly then subdivide into 150 mg packs, each of which shall have 5 mg atropine.

Q40. How would you weigh 12 mg of atropine with a maximum error of 5%, given a prescription balance whose sensitivity requirement is 6mg?	1. *Find the minimum weighable quantity:* $$\text{Smallest quantity weighable} = \frac{100 \times \text{Max. potential error}}{\text{Permissible \% error}}$$ $$= \frac{100 \times 6}{5} = 120 \; mg$$ 2. *Choose a pack of 150 mg, so that it contains the required 12 mg of atropine. The inert substance shall be 150 -12 -138 mg.* 3. *For 10 packs, the inert substance required = 138 x 10 = 1380 mg* *The active substance (atropine) required = 12 x 10 = 120 mg* *Total =1500 mg* *Mix the powders thoroughly. Weigh 150 mg and pack.* 4. *Each of the 150 mg Pack shall contain 12 mg Atropine and 138 mg Lactose.*
Q41. Supply 50 mg (+/- 5%) Chlorpheniramine maleate. The balance in the pharmacy has sensitivity requirement of 6 mg.	1. *Find the minimum weighable quantity:* $$\text{Smallest quantity weighable} = \frac{100 \times \text{Max. potential error}}{\text{Permissible \% error}}$$ $$= \frac{100 \times 6}{5} = 120$$ 2. *Choose a pack of 150 mg which shall contain 50 mg of chlorpheniramine and 100 mg of Lactose.* 3. *For 3 packs, the total amount required =* *Active ingredient = 50 x 3 = 150 mg* *Lactose = 100 x 3 = 300mg.*

Q42. A prescription balance has a sensitivity requirement of 6.5 mg. How will you weigh 20 mg of a substance with an error not greater than 2%?	Mix the powders thoroughly, weigh and pack 150 mg, that will contain 50 mg chlorpheniramine and 100 mg lactose 1. Calculate the minimum weighable quantity $= \dfrac{100 \times 6.5}{2} = 325$ mg 2. For convenience sake weigh 400 mg of the substance (which when divided into 20 packs, each shall have 20 mg of the substance. 3. Because the minimum weighable amount is 400 mg, each pack shall also weigh 400 mg, i.e. containing 20 mg active ingredient and 380 mg inert substance. 4. Total amount of inert substance = 380mg x 20 packs = 7600 mg Thus weigh 400 mg active substance, mix with 7600 mg inert substance, and pack in 400 mg packs.

General approach for preparation of aliquots:

EXAMPLE: Supply 20 mg Nifedipine within +/- 5% given a prescription balance with a sensitivity requirement of 6 mg.

Step 1: We cannot weigh 20 mg accurately. Therefore, we first determine the minimum weighable quantity according to the maximum potential error (= sensitivity requirement of a balance) and the permissible percent error:

$$Smallest\ quantity\ weighable = \frac{100 \times Max.\ potential\ error}{Permissible\ \%\ error}$$

$$= \frac{100 \times 6}{5} = 120\ mg$$

We can choose to weigh this amount or more but not less. In this example let us decide to weigh 120 mg of the drug Nifedipine.

Step 2: We need to set a predetermined weight of the drug-diluent mixture that will contain the amount of drug need, i.e. 20 mg nifedipine. This quantity must be equal to or greater than 120 mg, the minimum weighable weight. In this example we arbitrarily choose 150 mg. (we may decide to choose 120, or 180 or 200 mg or any other weight, as long as the weight is divisible, easily weighed and economical)

Step 3: Calculate the amount of the diluents need to be added to the drug, so that when we take 150 mg of the drug-diluent mixture, it will contain 20 mg nifedipine. The latter is calculated as follows:

$$\frac{20\ mg\ (drug\ needed\ in\ the\ prescription)}{150\ mg\ (drug - diluent\ mixture\ arbitrary\ chosen)} = \frac{120\ mg\ (total\ drug\ substance\ to\ be\ weighed)}{Y}$$

Where Y = total *drug-diluent* mixture to be prepared, from which we can deduce how much of the diluent is needed. In this case Y = 900 mg.

	Thus 900 *(total drug-diluent)* – 120 *(total drug)* = 780 *(diluent)*
	Amount of diluent to use = 780 mg. Answer.
Q43. A prescription balance has sensitivity requirement of 8 mg. Explain how you would weigh 12 mg of a substance with an error not greater than 5%	Determine the minimum weighable weight: $= \frac{100 \times 8}{5} = 160\ mg$
	Arbitrary choose to weigh 180 mg of the drug, if appropriate weights are available.
	Arbitrarily the weight of drug-diluent mixture is also chosen to be 180 mg.
	Calculate Y from the formula above:
	$$\frac{12}{180} = \frac{180}{Y}$$
	Y = 2700 mg
	The amount of diluents needed = 2700 – 180 = 2,520.
	Therefore, add 180 mg of the drug substance to 2,520 mg diluent and mix thoroughly. From this mixture if you take 180 mg, it will contain 12 mg of the active ingredient. (there will be such 15 packs
	[2700 ÷ 180 = 15]

3.4.2 Measurement of volume by aliquot method

Just like the case of solids above, some liquids such as dyes and very potent substances are needed in very minute quantities. The same principles used in the weighing minute quantities by aliquot method are employed in measurement of minute volumes of liquids.

Let us see how we can measure small volumes. Suppose you are asked to measure 1.25 milliliters of a dye solution. The only available measure is a pipette, which by all means you cannot measure 1.25 accurately. Therefore, we have to apply the aliquot method.

1. The first step is to select a multiple of the desired quantity that can be measured with the required accuracy and precision.

2. The second step is to dilute the quantity in (1) above with a compatible diluent to an amount evenly divisible by the multiple selected.

3. The final step is to measure the aliquot of the dilution that contains the quantity desired.

Step 1: Select the multiple of 1.25 mL. Let us select 4.
   This means that we can measure 6 mL (1.25mL x 4 = 6)
Step 2: Dilute the 6 mL in step 1 to 8 mL. Thus add 2 mL (6mL + 2 mL = 8 mL)
Step 3: Measure 1 mL of the dilution. This will contain 1.25 mL of the dye (this is because the original 6 mL of the dye is now contained in 8 mL. this means each mL contains $8 \div 6\ mL = 1.25\ mL$

NOTE we can select to measure 5 mL and dilute to 8 mL. 2 mL of the dilution shall contain 1.25 mL of the drug. [5 mL are in 8 mL. therefore 1.25 mL are contained in 2 mL]

Q44. Explain how you would obtain 0.5 mL of sulphuric acid using a 10 mL - pipette of 1 mL calibrations.	*4 is chosen as a multiple and the aliquot is set at 2 mL* *4 x 0.5 = 2 mL of the acid.* *Add 6 mL of the diluent to make 8 mL of the dilution so that measuring ¼ of the diluted solution (2 mL), 0.5 mL of the acid shall be obtained.* *Measure 2 mL of the acid. Dilute to 8 mL. Each 2 aliquot contains 0. 5 mL Answer*
Q45. Prepare a solution that will supply 0.6 mL of a dye. The tools you have include a 10 mL pipette of 1-mL graduations	*Step 1; choose a multiple. The most convenient multiple that will give a whole number is 5 (0.6 x 5 = 3 mL)* *Step 2. Select the volume of the aliquot. 2 mL is chosen. For a multiple of 5, the final volume will be 10 (2 x5 = 10 mL)* *Step 3: Measure 3 mL of the acid. Dilute to 10 mL with water. Take 2 mL of the diluted solution. This will contain 0.5 mL of the acid.*

CHAPTER 4

COMPUTATIONS IN METRIC SYSTEMS

4.1 Introduction

The process of converting a given value of volume, length or weight to a higher or lower denomination in called **Reduction**. When changing from a higher to lower denomination we call the process **Reduction descending**, while changing from lower to higher denomination is **reduction ascending**. In the metric system, one denomination is changed to another by simply moving the decimal point. It is a good habit to reduce a given quantity to the UNIT and then to the required denomination. Simply move a decimal point one place to the right to change a metric denomination to the next smaller one, OR move the decimal point one place to the left in order to change to the next larger denomination. The decimal point can be moved two, three or more places to the left or to the right depending on the reduction

Q 46.	Answers.
a. Reduce 5.62 kilograms to grams	a. $1\ kg = 10^3 g$ $5.62\ kg = 5.62 \times 10^3 g = 5620\ g$
b. Reduce 6548 milligrams to grams	b. $1\ mg = 10^{-3}\ g$ $6548\ mg = 6548 \times 10^{-3} = 6.548g$
c. Reduce 65 micrometers to centimeters	c. $1\ \mu m = 10^{-3}\ mm$ $65\ \mu m = 0.065\ mm$ $= 0.0065\ cm$
d. Complete the following:	
i. 350mg =.... g = ...kg = ... µ	i. $350\ mg = 0.35g = 0.00035kg = 350,000\ \mu g$
ii. 0.00045 mg = ... µg = ...ng = pg....	ii. $0.00045\ mg = 0.45\ \mu g = 450\ ng = 450,000 pg$
iii. 10mL = ... L = ... µL	iii. $10\ mL = 0.01L = 10,000\ \mu L$
iv. 30,000 µL = ... L = ... mL	iv. $30,000\ \mu L = 0.03L = 30\ mL$
v. 5088 µm = ...m =...cm = ...mm	v. $5088\ \mu m = 0.005088 m = 0.5\ cm = 5.088\ mm$

4.2 Addition and subtraction in metric systems:

To add or to subtract quantities in metric system, reduce them to a *common denominator* preferably the Unit of the table (i.e. Meter, liter or Gram) and arrange their denominate numbers for addition or subtraction. Note the position of the decimal point

| Q 47. How many grams do we get if we add 5 kg, 300 mg, and 750 g? | 5kg =   5,000   g
 300 mg =   0. 3 g
 750 g =   750 g
               5,750.3 g   Answer |

Q48. Add the following: 4.05g + 35,000 mg + 76,000,500 µg and express the answer in grams.	5.05 g = 5.05 g 35,000mg = 35 g 76,000,500 µg = 76.0005 g 116.0505 g Answer
Q49. 25.75 mm + 0.065 cm + 5080 µm = …mm	25.75 mm = 25.75 mm 0.065 cm = 65 mm 5080 µm = 5.080 mm 95. 830 mm
Q50. A sachet of powder contains 0.5 g of ingredient A, 0.05 g of ingredient B and 25 mg of ingredient C. What is the total weight in the sachet?	0.5 g = 0.5 g 0.05 g = 0.05 g 25 mg = 0.025 g Total = 0.575g
Q51. 112 mL + 0.75 L =	112 mL + 750 mL = 862 mL
Q52. A pharmacist withdrew 2.7L, 300 mL and 80 mL from a 5L container full of Alcohol. How much alcohol was left in the container?	Add the amount withdrawn: 2.7 L = 2.7 L 300 mL = 0.3 L 80mL = 0.08L 3.08L Subtract the total amount withdrawn from the initial amount in the container 5 L -3.08L 1. 92L Answer
Q53. A capsule contains the following amounts of ingredients: 0.355 g, 455 mg, 2.0 g and 900 mcg. Find the total weight of the ingredients.	0.355g = 0.355g 455 mg = 0.455g 2 g = 2g 900 mcg = 0.0009g 2.8109g =2810.9 mg
Q58. A pharmaceutical Assistant dispensed 320 mg and 450 mg of a drug from a container containing 10 g. How many grams were left in the container?	8. 320 mg +450 mg = 770 mg = 0.770 g 10 g – 0.770g = 9.230 g Answer

4.3 Multiplication and Division in metric systems

Every measurement in the metric system is expressed in single denomination. Computations therefore are done as discussed earlier in division and multiplication involving decimals. The product has the same denomination as the multiplicand. Likewise, the quotient has the same denomination as the dividend. Note the number of decimal places and allocate them accordingly in the multiplicand and quotient.

Multiply 3.5mL by 250:	250 X 3.5 750 1250 875.0 Answer

Divide 0.456g by 15:	$\phantom{15\sqrt{}}0.0304$ $15\sqrt{0.456}$ $\phantom{15\sqrt{0.}}\underline{45}$ $\phantom{15\sqrt{0.45}}60$ $\phantom{15\sqrt{0.45}}\underline{60}$ $\phantom{15\sqrt{0.45}}--$ *0.0304g Answer.*
multiply 55.5 mL by 45.66	55.5 x 45.66mL 2220 2775 3330 <u>3330</u> <u>2534.130</u> (There are three decimal places in the numbers which are multiplied)

CHAPTER 5

Apothecary and Avoirdupois Systems Compared to Metric System.

5.1 Introduction.

The units of measure and weight of the Avoirdupois and Apothecary systems although sharing the same names, they differ in values. The only denomination common to both systems is weight unit known as *"grain"*.

The word **avoirdupois** is from Anglo-Norman French *aveir de peis* (later *avoir de pois*), literally "goods of weight". It is a system of weights that was used in the United States, Canada and later in United Kingdom (including British colonies) before the Metric system was adopted. Weight is almost always expressed in avoirdupois system. In Avoirdupois system the ounce is equal to 437.7 grains while the pound is 16 ounces. The **Apothecary system (imperial system)** is a system of weights used in pharmacy and based on an ounce equal to 480 grains and a pound equal to 12 ounces. It has been largely replaced by measures of the metric system.

Pharmacists used to buy drugs by avoirdupois weight and sold them by apothecary weight. The apothecary pound is 1240 grains lighter than the avoirdupois pound, whereas the apothecary ounce is 42.5 heavier than the avoirdupois ounce. However, when compounding prescriptions, pharmacists employ apothecaries' and metric system to weigh and measure ingredients.

5.2 The Apothecaries' System

1. Weight

20 grains (gr)	=	1 scruple (Ə)
3 scruples (60 grains)	=	1 drachm(ʒ)) = 60 grains
8 drams (480grains)	=	1 ounce (℥) = 480 grains
12 ounces (5760 grains)	=	1 pound (lb.)

The table may also be represented as:

lb	ʒ	℥	Ə	gr
1	12	96	288	5760
	1	8	24	480
		1	3	60
			1	20

2. Volume

60 minims (♏)) =	1 fluid drachm or dram (f ʒ)
8 fluids drams' f ʒ =1 fluid ounce (f℥)	
16 fluid ounces f℥ = 1 Pint (pt)	
2 pints (32 fluid ounces) = 1 quart (qt)	
4 quarts (8pints) 1 gallon	

This table may also be presented as

gal	qt	pt	f℥	f ʒ	♏
1	4	8	128	1024	61440
	1	2	32	256	15360
		1	16	128	7680
			1	8	480
				1	60

Avoirdupois measure of weight
437.5 (or 437 ½) grain (gr) = 1 ounce (oz)
16 ounces (7000 grains) = 1 pound (lb)

lb	oz	gr
1	16	7000
	1	437.5

Note that whereas the **apothecary ounce is 480 grains**, the **Avoirdupois ounce is 437.5 grains**. Also **apothecary pound is 12 ounces** and therefore 12 x 480 grains = 5760 grains while the **avoirdupois pound is 16 ounce** and therefore 16 x 437.5 grains = 7000 grains.

And to facilitate the interpretation of these prescriptions, the relationships and conversion factors contained herein **MUST BE MEMORISED**.

The length was measured in terms of inches, feet, yards, furlongs and miles.

5.3 FUNDAMENTAL COMPUTATIONS IN AVOIRDUPOIS AND APOTHECARY SYSTEMS

It is important to note that when using these systems, the amount is usually expressed in short using Latin abbreviations. The common abbreviations used are

1. ss or s̄s̄ = one half
2. i = 1
3. ii = 2
4. iii = 3
5. iv = 4

The values in Common Systems are recorded in Compound quantities (that is mixed quantities) and therefore when dealing with them you must do *simplification* by reducing the quantity to a compound quantity. Minims and grains are not expressed as decimals but rather by fractions;

Q59. Reduce ℥ ss ʒ ii ℈ii to grains	Interpretation: Reduce one half of an ounce, two drachms and two minims to grains. Calculation: ℥ss = 0.5 x 480gr = 240 gr ʒii = 2 x 60 grains = 120 gr ℈ii = 2 x 20 grain = 40 gr 400 gr.
Q60. Reduce f℥iv f℥iisspt i to fluiddrams	Interpretation: Reduce four fluidounces, 2 ½ fluidrams and one pint to fluid drams Calculation: f℥iv = 4 x 8 = 32 fluid dram ℥iss = 2 ½ fluid dram pt = 1 x 16 x 8 = 128 fluidram 162 ½ fluidrams
To **add** or to **subtract** quantities in the Common system, reduce the result to a compound quantity **Q61.** Add 4 pounds, 4 ounces, 2 drams and 60 grains to 5 pounds, 7 ounces, 4 drams, 6 grains (apothecary)	lb. ℥ ʒ gr 4 4 2 60 5 7 4 6 9 11 6 66 But 11 ounces = 1 lb. +3 ounces. Thus add 1 lb. to lb. column 66 grains = 1 drams + 6 grains. Thus add 1 ʒ to ʒ column **The Answer is 10 lb. 3 ounces 7 drams and 6 grains.**
Q62. Add the following volumes: 6 gals, 3 pt, 3 fl oz and 2 pt, 2fl oz, 4 fl dr	Properly arrange the volumes sequentially starting from biggest to lowest left to rightwise; then compute and where necessary reduce larger quantities to smaller ones: Gal pt fl oz fl dr 6 3 3 2 2 4 6 5 5 4

	But 1 qt = 2 pt, hence 5 pt = 2qt + 1 pt
	6 gals, 6 pt, 2 qt, 1 pt, 5 fl oz and 4 fl dr Answer.
Q63. You have 2 gal of a medicine. If you withdraw 1 pt, 4 fl oz and 6 fl dr from the 2 gal how much do you remain with?	Divide 1 gal into 4 qt, leaving 1 gal into its column; divide one of the 4 qt into 2 pt, leaving 3 qt; divide 1 pt into 16 fl oz, leaving 1 fl oz; divide 1 fl oz into 8 fl dr leaving 15 fl oz

Gal	qt	pt	fl oz	fl dr
1	3	1	15	8
		1	4	6
1	3	0	11	2

The answer is 1 gal, 3qt 11fl oz and 2 fl dr

5.3.1 Multiplication of common system

Remember: 8 fl dr = 1 fl oz
16 fl oz = 1 pt
2 pt = 1 qt
4 qt = 1 gal
LEARN THESE BY HEART

Q 64. multiply 3pt, 5 fl oz, 6 fl dr by 6	*Arrange the quantities in the descending order of magnitude towards the right and multiply. The products have the same denomination as the multiplicand. Multiply fractions as usual. Reduce larger quantities to smaller ones.*

pt	fl oz	fl dr
3	5	6
		X 6
18	30	36

(i)   36 fl dr = 3 fl oz + <u>6 fl dr</u>
(ii) 30 fl oz + 3 fl oz (from (i)) = 33 fl oz = 2 pt + <u>1 fl oz</u>
(iii) 18 pt + 2 pt (from (ii) = 20 pt = 10 qt = 2 gals + <u>2 qt</u>

THE ANSWER IS **2 gal 2 qt 1 fl oz 2 pt and 6 fl dr**

Q 65. A formula calls for 1 pt 4 fl oz, 5 fl dr of Oils. How much of each oil do you need if you are to prepare four times the amount in the formula?	pt	fl oz	fl dr
	1	5	5
			X 4
	4	20	20

(i)   20 fl dr = 2 fl oz + 4 fl dr
(ii) 20 fl oz + 2 fl oz (from (i) = 24 fl oz = 1 pt + 8 fl oz
(iii) 4 pt = 1 gal

THE ANSWER IS *1 gal 1 pt 8 fl oz and 4 fl dr*

5.3.2 Division

The quotient always has the same denomination as the dividend. If the dividend has different denominations, arrange as in Multiplication above, begin division with the largest quantity at the left, convert the reminder, if any, into the next lower units and add to the next column before proceeding with the division. Fractions are treated just like in multiplication.

Q 66. Divide 12gal, 3 pt, 8 fl oz by 6 $6\sqrt{\begin{array}{ccc} \text{Gal} & \text{pt} & \text{fl oz} \\ 12 & 3 & 8 \end{array}}$	12 gal ÷ 6 = 2 gal 3 pt = 48 fl oz. Add this to the available 8 fl oz. = 48+8 = 56. Thus $\frac{56}{6} = 9\frac{2}{6} = 9\frac{1}{3}$ = 9 fl oz and 1/3 fl oz 1/3 fl oz = 8 x 1/3 fluid drams = 2 fl dr and 2/3 o fl dr 2/3 fl dr = 2/3 x 60 minims = 40 minims **The answer** is 2 gal 9 fl oz 2 fl dr and 40 Minims. You can also reduce all quantities to the small unit (fl oz in this example: (12 gal x 128 fl oz) + (3 pt x 16 fl oz) + (8 fl oz) = 1536 + 48 + 8 = 1592 fl oz 1592 fl oz ÷ 6 = $265\frac{2}{6}$ fl oz OR $265\frac{1}{3}$ fl oz Extract the largest units possible: In this case the biggest unit is 128 fl oz in one gallon, and twice this figure is possible: 265 − 128 x2 (equivalent to two gallons) = 265 − 256 = 9 fl oz
Q67. How many capsules of 15 minims each can be obtained from 20 fl oz of active ingredient?	As above, $\frac{1}{3}$ fl oz = 2 fl dr and 40 minims. 1 fl oz = 480 minims 20 fl oz = 9600 minims Number of capsules = 9600 ÷15 = **640 capsules**. Answer.
Q68. How many tablets containing 0.05 gr can be made from 2 gr?	$\frac{2gr}{0.05}$ =2gr / 0.05 = **40 tablets**. Answer

5.4 Household measures

Liquid medicines are sometimes prescribed to be taken at home in quantities which one may not be able to measure accurately. This may be so because a specific measure for that volume is not available. Since time immemorial, there have been "household measures" used to estimate the volume to be taken. Customarily the household measures are estimated as follows.

1 tumblerful	= f℥ viii (8 fluidounces)	= 240 mL
1 teacup	= f℥ iv (4 fluidounces)	= 120 mL
1 wineglass	= f℥ii (2 fluidounces)	= 60 mL
2 tablespoonsful	= f℥ i (1 fluidounce)	= 30 mL
1 tablespoonful	= f ʒiv (4 fluiddrachm)	= 15 mL (= ½ fluidounce)
1 dessertspoonful	= f ʒii (2 fluiddrachm)	= 8 mL
*1 teaspoonful	= f ʒI (1 fluiddrachm)	= 5 mL
½ teaspoon	= f ʒ ss ½ fluiddrachm)	= 2 mL (or 2.5 mL)

*The volume of a teaspoon is controversial. USP consider it to be 5 mL, while other prescribers consider it to be 4 mL. However, there is no standard teaspoon and household teaspoon have capacities varying from 3 to 7 mL, while tablespoons vary from 15 to 22 mL.

Frequently a "drop" is used as a measure for medicines, especially when administering very small quantities. But the volume of fluids depends on many factors including density, viscosity, surface tension, temperature and shape and nature of surface of a "dropper". Thick viscous fluid (e.g. n ad syrups will have large volumes while mobile liquids with high density and little adhesion to dropper surface will have considerably smaller volume. A "standard dropper" according to pharmacopeias is 3 mm in external diameter at its delivery end and when held vertically at 25C, it delivers 20 drops of water per mL. thus each drop is estimated at 45 – 55 mg or averagely 0.05 mL.

CHAPTER 6

CONVERSION OF METRIC /COMMON/METRIC SYSTEMS

6.1 Introduction.

Metric system is almost entirely predominating in use in pharmacy. Most prescriptions and medication orders are written in metric systems. Doses are expressed in metric units. The Common system is almost replaced. However there are times when one may come across a prescription written in Common units, or you may be called upon to translate an order or a formular expressed in old Common system. The balance in use may have weights in Common system. You MUST be able to perform a conversion from metric to Common system and vice versa.

When it is required to do a conversion, a single system must be adopted, and reduced to a common denomination. Subsequently, a *conversion factor* is required to change one denomination in one system into another.

For practical purposes, the following table should provide you with quick conversion factors in weight, volume and length and these **conversions** or interrelationships MUST BE MEMORISED. Also it is suggested that tables of equivalents be kept in a conspicuous and convenient place in the Prescription or Compounding Department.

Table 3 Metric-Avoirdupios interconversions.

WEIGHT		VOLUME		LENGTH	
1 g	15.432 gr	1 mL	16.23 ♏	1 m	39.37 in
1 kg	2.20 lb	1 ♏ (minim)	0.06 mL	1 in	2.54 cm
1 gr	0.065g (or 65mg)	1 f ʒ	3.69 mL	1 in	25 mm
1 oz (avoir)	28.35 g	1 f ℥	29.57 mL	1 μm	1/1000 mm
1 ʒ	31.1 g	1 pt	473 mL	1 μm	1/25,000 in
1 lb (avoir)	454 g	1 gal(US)	3785 mL		
1 lb (apoth)	373.2 g				

Other equally useful conversion factors are :

    1 oz (avoir) = 437.5 gr
    1 ʒ = 480 gr
    1 gal (U.S.) = 128 ℥
    1 ℥ (water) = 455 gr

Question	Conversion	Solution
Q 69. Convert 3 fluidounces to milliliters	1 f℥ = 29.57 mL	Multiply the number of fluidounces by 29.57 $3 \times 29.57 = 88.71\ mL$ This can also be done by proportions: $$\frac{1\ (f℥)}{3((f℥))} = \frac{29.57\ (mL)}{x(mL)}$$ $x = 88.71\ mL$
Q70. Convert 5 mL to fluidounces	1 f℥ = 29.57 mL	Divide the number of mL by 29.57 $5 \div 29.57 = 0.17\ f℥$ Or by proportions: $$\frac{1(f℥)}{x(f℥)} = \frac{29.57\ (mL)}{5\ (mL)}$$ $x = 0.17\ f℥$
Q71. A cough syrup contained 1/8 gr of pholcodin per teaspoonful (5 mL). How much pholcodin would be needed to prepare 1 ½ pint of the syrup?	1 pt = 473 mL	1 ½ pt = 1 ½ x 473 mL = 709.5 mL There is 1/8 gr in 5 mL. How many grains are in 709.5 mL? $$\frac{1/8\ gr}{x\ gr} = \frac{5\ mL}{709.5\ mL}$$ $x = \frac{709.5\ x\ 1/8}{5} = 17.7\ gr$ Answer
Q 72. How many liters are equal to 3 gal and 25 f℥?	1 gal(US) = 3785 mL = 3.785 L 1 f℥ = 29.57 mL	3 gal = 3 x 3.785 L = 11.355 L 25 f℥ = 25 x 29.57 mL = 739.25 mL = 0.739 L Total volume = 11.355 L + 0.739 L = 12.1 L Answer.
Q73. A piece of gauze measures 12.5 mm. Express this in inches	12.5 mm = 1.25 cm 1 in = 2.54 cm	Divide the number of centimeters by 2.54 $1.25\ cm = \frac{1.25}{2.54}\ inches = 0.49\ in$ Or by proportion: $\frac{1\ (in)}{x(in)} = \frac{2.54\ cm}{1.25\ cm}$ $x =$ 0.49 in. Answer.
Q74. A tile measures 15 inches by 12 inches. Put these dimensions in metric system. Express the area of the tile in square meters.	1 in = 2.54 cm	Multiply the number of inches by 2.54 15 x 2.54 cm = 38.1 cm or 0.381 m 12 x 2.54 cm = 30.48 cm or 0.3048 m The area = 0.381 x 0.3048 = 0.12 m^2 Ans. (Note that the answer is given to 2 decimal places)

Q75. A mercury barometer reads pressure as 760 mm of Mercury. How many inches are they/	1 in =2.54 cm = 25.4 mm	760 mm = 760/25 inches = 30.4 inches
	If conversion factor "1 in = 25 mm" is used, the answer is significantly different!!	$\dfrac{760\ mm}{25.4\ mm} = \dfrac{x\ inches}{1\ inches}$ $x = 760/25 = 29.9\ inches$ ** Note the difference due to approximation of 2.54 to 2.5!! The accurate conversion factor is 1 in = 2.54 cm. When the length is short, approximation "1 in = 25 mm" can be used.
Q76. How many minims are in 5 mL	1 mL = 16.23 ℳ	$5mL = 5 \times 16.23\ ℳ = 81.15\ ℳ$
Q77. How many fluidounces are found in 3L?	1 f℥ = 29.57 mL 3 L = 3000 mL	$\dfrac{1(f℥)}{x(f℥)} = \dfrac{29.57\ (mL)}{3000\ (mL)}$ $x = 101.45\ f℥$ Answer.
Q78. How many mL are equivalent to fℨiiss?	fℨiiss = 2½ fℨ 1 fℨ =3.69 mL	Multiply the number of fluiddrachms by 3.69 $2\ ½\ fℨ \times 3.69 = 9.23\ mL$
Q79. How many grains (apoth) are equivalent to 16 grams?	1g = 15.432 gr	$\dfrac{1\ gram}{16\ grams} = \dfrac{15.432}{x}$ $x = 246.912\ gr$ Answer. Or simply multiply the number of gram by 15.432
Q80. Convert 25 mg to grains	1 gr = 65 mg (or 1gr =0.065 g)	$\dfrac{1\ gr}{x\ gr} = \dfrac{65\ mg}{25\ mg}$ $x = \dfrac{25}{65} = \dfrac{5}{13}\ gr = 0.38\ gr$
Q81. Convert 12kg to pounds (avoir.)	1 lb (avoir) =454 g =0.454 kg	$\dfrac{1\ lb}{x\ lb} = \dfrac{0.454\ kg}{12\ kg}$ $= 26.4\ lb$
	OR 1 kg = 2.2 lb	$12kg = 12 \times 2.2\ lb = 26.4\ lb$ Answer.
Q82. How many grams are equivalent to 7.25 gr?	1 gr = 65 mg	$7.25\ gr = 65 \times 7.25\ g = 471.25\ mg$
Q83. Bricanyl® inhaler canister for treatment of astma releases 500 mcg per inhalation. How many grains are inhaled?	1 gr = 65 mg = 65,000 mcg	$\dfrac{1\ gr}{x\ gr} = \dfrac{65,000\ mcg}{500\ mcg}$ $x = 0.008\ gr$ Answer.

Q84. Codein Linctus has 15 mg codeine sulphate per 5 mL. Express this concentration in gr per minims	1 gr = 65 mg 1 mL = 16.23 ℳ.	15 mg = 15/65 gr = 0.23 gr 5 mL = 5 x 16.23 ℳ = 81.15 ℳ Therefore, 15 mg per 5 mL = 0.23 gr per 81.15 ℳ This can further be simplified to $$\frac{0.23\ gr}{x\ gr} = \frac{81.15\ ℳℳ}{1\ ℳℳ}$$ x = 0.23/81.15 = 0.003 or 0.003 gr per Minim
Q85. f℥ i of Methadone syrup (as used in treatment of cough in terminal illness), contains 10 gr methadone. How many mg of methadone are in 5 mL of the syrup?	f℥i = one fluid ounce, (1 fl oz) = 30 mL Also 1 gr = 65 mg	There are 10 gr in 1 fl oz. Therefore there are 10 x 65 mg in 1 fl oz. = 650 mg in 1 fl oz Therefore there are 650 mg in 30 mL $$\frac{650\ mg}{x\ mg} = \frac{30\ mL}{5\ mL}$$ $x = \frac{5 \times 650}{30} = 108.33$ or 108 mg per mL

CHAPTER 7

CALCULATIONS INVOLVING DENSITY AND SPECIFIC GRAVITY

7.1 Introduction.

Different substances with equal volume have diferent weights. For example cotton is less heavy compared to a stone having the same volume as cotton. It is easy to carry a plastic than to carry a piece of steel iron having the same volume. A 20 liter pail containing paint is heavier compared to the same pail containg water.

In pharmaceutical compounding we weigh ingredients in order to mix and make prescribed preparations. Viscous ingredients are weighable but difficult to transfer without losing some amount that stick in the container where the substance was weighed. But with the knowledge of its weight per certain volume, we can measure the volume of a particulr weight.

Density and specific gravity are terms that used to express relative weights of equal volumes of substances. Density is defined as Mass per unit volume of a substance, usually expressed as grams per cubic centimeter (g/cm^3) or grams per milliliter (g/mL). Mathematically, it expressed as :

$$\text{Density} = \frac{mass\ (grams)}{volume\ (mL)}$$

Q86. 100 mL of sulphuric acid weigh 180 g. Calculate its density.	Desity $=\frac{mass}{volume} = \frac{180\ g}{100\ mL} = 1.8\ g\ per\ mL$

Specific gravity is the ratio of the mass of a substance to the mass of an equal volume of another substance taken as a standard, at the same temperature and pressure. In pharmacy, the standard substance is water.

$$\text{Specific gravity} = \frac{weight\ of\ a\ given\ volume\ of\ a\ substance}{weight\ of\ an\ equal\ volume\ of\ water}$$

Specific gravity is a ratio of like quantities and hence has no units or dimensions. It is more convenient to use specific gravity than density, because specific gravity has no variations. Whereas the density of water is 1 g/cm^3, 455 grains/fluidounce or 62 ½ pounds per cubic feet, specific gravity (s.g.) is always 1.

7.2 Calculations involving densities and specific gravities

Q87. Calculate the specific gravity of Sunflower oil if 500 mL weigh 485 g	500 mL of water weigh 500 g Specific gravity of the oil = $\frac{weight\ of\ oil}{weight\ of\ an\ equal\ volume\ of\ water} = \frac{485}{500} = 0.97$
Q88. Copper having a volume of 9 cubic centimeter, weighs 80.4 g. Calculate its s.g.	9 c.c of water weigh 9 g s.g $=\frac{80.4}{9} = 8.93$
Q89. 450 mL of linseed oil weigh 390 g. Calculate tits specific gavity	The weight of an equal volume of water (450mL) is 450 g. Thefore specific gravity =

$$\frac{weight\ of\ linseed\ oil}{weight\ of\ equal\ volume\ of\ water} = \frac{390}{450} = 0.87$$

Specific gravity, weight and volume of a substance are interrelated and when two of the three factors are known, a third factor can be easily calculated. When given specific gravity of a substance and its volume you can find its its weight. Likewise you can determine the volume of a liquid given its specific gravity and its weight.

$$\frac{specific\ gravity\ of\ water}{specific\ gravity\ of\ a\ liquid} = \frac{weight\ of\ an\ equal\ volume\ of\ water}{X}$$

Where X is the weight of the liquid. Specific gravity of water is 1. Therefore,

Weight of a liquid = $\frac{(weight\ of\ an\ equal\ volume\ of\ water) \times (specific\ gravity\ of\ a\ liquid)}{1}$

Weight of the liquid = Specific gravity of the liquid x weight of an equal volume of water

(because the specific gravity of water is One, its weight in grams = its volume in mL)

[Wt = s.g. x volume]

Volume of the liquid = $\frac{volume\ of\ equal\ weight\ of\ water}{specific\ gravity\ of\ the\ liquid}$

(because the specific gravity of water is 1, volume of an equal weight of water is equal to the weight of the liquid)

$$[volume = \frac{weight}{specific\ gravity}]$$

Q90. What is the weight of 150 mL of sulphuric acid? (specific gravity of sulphuric acid = 1.84)	Wt = s.g. x volume = 1.84 x 150 = 276 g
Q91. Specific gravity of alcohol is 0.812. what is the weight in kilograms of 9 liters of alcohol?	9 liters = 9000 mL Weight = s.g X volume = 0.812 x 9000 = 7308 g = 7.308kg
Q92. Chloroform has specific gravity of 1.475. How much do 3.5 liters of chloroform weigh?	3.5 L = 3500 mL Weight = s.g. X v = 1.475 X 3500 = 5162.5 g = 5.16 kg
Q93. 500 mL of liquid paraffin are required to prepare 1 liter of a mineral oil emulsion. How many grams of liquid paraffin would be needed to prepare 6 liters of the emulsion? (s.g of liq. Paraffin = 0.87)	Total volume of liquid paraffin required = 500 mL per liter x 6 liters = 500 x 6= 3000 mL Weight = s.g x v = 0.87 x 3000 = 2610 g = 2.6 kg.
Q94. Glycerin has specific gravity 1.2. What is the volume of glycerin that weighs 56 g?	$s.g = \frac{weight\ of\ liquid}{weight\ of\ equal\ volume\ of\ water}$ therefore weight of equal volume of water $= \frac{weight\ of\ liquid}{specigic\ gravity\ of\ liqiquid} = \frac{56}{1.2}$

	=46.67g. But for all practical purpose, the weight of water in grams = volume of water in mL

Thus the volume of water and hence the volume of glycerin = 46.67 mL |
| Q95. What is the volume of 900 g of mercury (s.g. 13.6) | Volume = weight/specific gravity = $\frac{900}{13.6}$ = 66.18 mL |
| Q96. 350 g of chloroform (s.g. 1.575) and 1.65 kg of methylsalicylate ((s.g. 1.180) were mixed too make a liniment. What is the volume of the resulting solution? | Volume of chloroform = $\frac{350}{1.575}$ = 222.22 mL
Volume of mehtl salicylate = $\frac{1650\,(mL)}{1.18}$ = 916.67 mL
Total volume (assuming no contraction or expansion on mixing) = 222.22 + 916.76 = 1138.9 mL Answer. |
| Q97. 60 glycerin suppositories are made using the following formula:
Glycerin   90 g
  Sodium stearate   10 g
  Purified water   10 mL

Calculate the volume of glycerin required to make 15 suppositories given that the specific gravity of glycerin is 1.25 | 60 suppositorries require 90 grams. Let us calculate how many gams are required to make 15 suppositories:
$\frac{90\,g}{X\,g} = \frac{60\,suppositories}{15\,suppositorie}$ $X = \frac{15 \times 90}{60}$ = 22.5 g

If s.g. is 1.25, then the volume of glycerin required
= $\frac{weight}{s.g.}$ = $\frac{22.5}{1.25}$ = 18 mL Answer |
| Q98. ℞ Mouth rinse
Sig 15 mL tid 2/52
The formular of the mouth rinse is 1.6 mL Cinnamon oil in enough water to make 1000 mL solution.

a) What weight of cinammon oil is required? (s.g. of cinnamon oil is 1.050) | Total volume of cinnamon oil mouthwash required = 15 mL x 3 times a day x 14 days (2 weeks) = 630 mL
For 1000mL we need 1.6 mL, thus for 650 mL we need
$\frac{1000}{650} = \frac{1.6}{X}$ $X = 1.04\,mL$

Weight of 1.04 mL cinnamon oil = s.g. x volume
= 1.050 x 1.04
= 1.092g (approx 1.1 g) |
| b) Cinnamon oil costs 150,000.00 shillings per kilo. How much shall we pay if we make 50 liters of the mouth wash? | Each liter needs 1.6 mL. Therefore 50 liter shall require
50 x 1.6 mL = 80 mL
The weight of 80 mL cinnamon = s.g. x volume
= 1.050 x 80
= 84g

1 kg (1000 mL) costs 150,000 Shillings. We need to calculate how much 84 mg shall cost:

$\frac{1000}{84} = \frac{150,000}{x}$ $X = 12,600$ Shillings. Answer. |

7.3 Measurement of Specific Gravity

Specific gravity is measured by using specific gravity bottle (or a pycnometer), a hydrometer or a westphal balance. Let us see an example of how specific gravity bottle may be used to determine s.g. of a substance. (The reader is refered elsewhere for practical application and determination of specific gravities using the other instruments).

The specific gravity bottle is weighed empty first. Then it is weighed when filled with water. Finally it is weighed when filled with a liquid whose specific gravity is to be determined. Using this bottle the volume of water and the liquid are equal. Specific gravity is computed as

Specific Gravity = $\frac{weight\ of\ bottle\ with\ liquid - weight\ of\ empty\ bottle}{weight\ og\ bottle\ with\ water - weight\ of\ empty\ bottle}$

A pycnometer is a container intended to determine the specific gravity of liquid substance. It has a specified capacity or volume, usually 10, 20, or 30 mL.

Q99. A pycnometer weighs 23.5 g when empty. When filled with water it weighs 48.4 g. When filled with another liquid, it weighs 49.8. Find the specific gravity of the liquid	$\frac{49.8 - 23.5}{48.4 - 23.5} = 1.068$ Answer.

CHAPTER 8

CALCULATION OF DOSES

8.1 terminologies used in posology.

Posology is the branch of medical science that deals with the doses of drugs and their preparations. The knowledge of this subject is of utmost importance for pharmacy practitioners, doctors and nurses.

Dose in pharmacy is defined as the quantitative amount of medicine administered or taken by patient for the intended medicinal effect. Less than this amount is **Underdose** and more than this amount is **Overdose**.

A dose may be **single dose**, whereby the amount is taken at one time. For example, in the treatment of malaria, two (2) metakelfin® (a trade name for Sulphadoxine and Pyrimethamine) tablets are taken as a single dose. But the dose could be administered in a **multidose** or **daily dose**. For instance, two capsules each containing 250 mg amoxicillin, are taken eight hourly for five consecutive days to treat upper respiratory infection. The total amount taken during the time-course therapy is the **total dose.** In the case of amoxicillin, the total dose for treating upper respiratory tract infection is 500 mg x 3 times a day x 5 days = 7500 mg or 7.5 g, the schedule of dosing (for example four time a day for two weeks) is known as **Dosage Regimen.**

The dose of a drug is determined by various aspects. Thus the dose may be given once daily or several times a day depending on

1. The chemical and pharmacological activity of the medicine,
2. Physical and chemical characteristics of the medicine
3. The dosage form in which the medicine is administered (e.g. tablet, sustained release formulation, injection, or inhalation)
4. The route of administration (oral, injection, topical application, intramuscular or intravenous injection)
5. Patients' characteristics (age, body weight, body surface area, disease condition and its severity, liver and kidney function)

The amount of medicine which may be expected ordinarily to produce the intended effect in an adult person is known as **the usual dose.** This is the amount upon which all other doses are modified to suit individual patients, such as infants (**Pediatric dose),** children (**Child dose**), and special patient groups e.g. patients with renal or kidney failure.

It is important when you are filling the prescription or dispensing to check if the dose is correct. This is the responsibility of the dispenser more than that of a prescriber. Pharmacists carry a legal responsibility in ensuring the correct dose, short of which may lead to prosecution on the basis of professional negligence. Should you find the dose to be unusual, you are ethically bound to consult the prescriber to ensure that the dose is as intended and is correct?

In the process of compounding, you should be able to calculate the total amount of ingredients needed in compounding according to the formula given. When dispensing medicines, you should be able to find out the exact volume of liquid medicines (such as syrups, solutions, emulsion and suspensions) to be supplied for a given period of time. For solid dosage form, you should be able to determine the number of capsules or tablets to be supplied according to the prescription.

Formulae for calculation of doses.

1. $Number\ of\ doses = \dfrac{Total\ Amount}{Size\ of\ dose}$

2. $Size\ of\ dose = \dfrac{total\ amount}{Number\ of\ doses}$

3. Total amount = Number of doses × Size of dose

4. $Quantity\ in\ each\ dose = \dfrac{Quantity\ in\ total\ amount}{Number\ of\ doses}$

5. When the number of doses is not given,

$$\dfrac{Total\ amount}{Size\ of\ dose} = \dfrac{(Quantity\ in\ total\ amount)}{x}$$

Where x is the unknown quantity in each dose.

8.1 Calculations of doses.

8.1.1. To Calculate the quantity of ingredients needed to make a given amount or volume of medicine according to the formula given.	*The prescription calls for compounding 60 mL of codeine Linctus NP. The formula given is for making 1000 mL*
e.g. M. ft. 60mL Codeine Linctus NP.	*How much of each of the ingredients are required in 60 mL?*
Interpretation Mix and make 60 codeine Linctus NP	*We must calculate the* $\dfrac{quantity\ required}{total\ amount\ of\ the\ medicine\ in\ the\ formula}$
According to the National Pharmacopoeia (NP), the formula for codeine Linctus is as follows:	*This is* $\dfrac{60}{1000} = 0.06$. *This is also known as the conversion factor.*
Codeine PO₄ 3 g Lemon syrup 200 mL Benzoic Acid solution 20 mL Water 20 mL Cod Tartrazine solution 10 mL Syrup, to 1000 mL	*Each ingredient is thus multiplied by the conversion factor 0.06 to get the required amount of each ingredient.* Codeine PO₄ 3 g x 0.06 =0.18 g = **180 mg** Lemon syrup 200 mL x 0.06 = **12 mL** Benzoic Acid solution 20 mL x 0,06= **1.2 mL** Water 20 mL x 0.06= **1.2 mL** Cpd Tartrazine solution 10 mL x 0.06= **0.6 mL** Syrup, to **60mL**

Q110.
℞. M ft. Noscapine Linctus
    Sig. ii tsp qid x 5/7
Calculate the amount of Noscapine required in this prescription.
 	
Look up for the formula of Noscapine Linctus. The TPH give the formula as follows:
  Noscapine   0.3 g
  Citric acid monohydrate   1.0 g
  Cpd Tartraxine Soln   0.3 mL
  Chloroform spirit   7.5 mL
  Water for Prep.   10 mL
  Syrup Ad   100 mL
	1 tsp (teaspoon) = 5 mL. Thus 2 tsp = 10 mL
	
	Total amount required = 10 mL four times a day for five days
	
	= 10 x 4 x 5 = 200 mL.
	
	According to the formula, there are 0.3 g in 100 mL. How many are required in 200 mL?
	
	By ratio: $\frac{100\ mL}{200\ mL} = \frac{0.3\ g}{x\ g}$ x= 0.6g Answer

8.1.2 To calculate the number of doses in a given volume of the medicine:

$$\text{The number of doses} = \frac{\text{total amount}}{\text{Size of Dose}}$$

Q101. The dose of digoxin is 125 mcg. How many doses are contained in 1.5 g digoxin	The number of doses = $\frac{\text{total amount}}{\text{Size of Dose}}$ 1.5 g = 1500000 mcg Number of doses = $\frac{1500000\ mg}{125\ mg}$ = 12000 doses. Answer
Q102. The dose of iron sulphate required to rectify anemia is 200 mg daily. How many doses can be made from 5 g iron sulphate	Use formula number 1 above: **Number of doses** = $\frac{\text{total amount}}{\text{Size of Dose}}$ 5 g = 5,000 mg Number of doses = $\frac{5,000\ (mg)}{200\ (mg)}$ = 25 doses. Answer
Q103. 100 mLs of a syrup have been dispensed to a patient who was instructed to take it in a dose of 2 teaspoonfuls three times a day. How many teaspoonfuls will the patient get?	1 teaspoonful is estimated to be 5 mL. **Number of teaspoonfuls** = $\frac{\text{total amount}}{\text{size of dose}} = \frac{100\ mL}{5\ mL}$ = 20 tsp. Answer

8.1.3 To calculate the size of each dose in a given quantity of medicine and the number of doses it contains:

$$Size\ of\ dose = \frac{total\ amount}{Number\ of\ doses}$$

Q104. What is the volume of a dose if 200mL of Metoclopramide were to be given in 14 doses? How many teaspoonfuls should be given for each dose?	There are 200 mL to be given in 14 doses. $The\ size\ of\ each\ dose = \frac{total\ amount}{number\ of\ doses}$ $= \frac{200}{14} = 14.3 = Aprox.\ 14\ mL$ Each teaspoonful is approximately 5mL. Therefore, in 14 mL there are approx. 3 teaspoonfuls. Thus the patient should be given 3 teaspoonfuls in 14 doses.
Q105. 10 mL of Neomycin eye drops 5% are to be administered in 40 doses. How many drops should be given?	A pharmaceutical dropper has approx. 32 drops per mL. Thus in 10 mL there are 10 x 32 drops = 320 drops $Size\ of\ dose = \frac{total\ amount}{number\ of\ doses}$ $= \frac{320\ drops}{40\ (doses)} = 8\ drops,\ Answer.$
Q106. Codeine cough syrup contains 240 mg of codeine phosphate in 0.12 L. How many mgs are contained in each teaspoonful of the syrup?	240 mg are contained in 0.12 L or 120 mL of syrup. A teaspoonful is 5 mL. By proportion: $\frac{240mL}{120mL} = \frac{x\ mg}{5mg}$ therefore $x = \frac{5 \times 240}{120}$ x = 10 mg Answer.

8.1.4 To calculate the total amount of medicine, given how many doses and the size of each dose:

$$Total\ amount = (number\ of\ doses) \times (size\ of\ dose)$$

Q107. How many mL of a medicine would be taken in total at a dose of two tablespoonful's twice a day for one week?	Number of tablespoonful's (the dose) = 2tbsp x 2 times a day x 7 days = 2 x 2 x 7 = 28 Each tablespoon carries 15 mL. Total amount of medicine = Number of doses x size of each dose = 28 x 15 = 420 mL.
Q108. Paracetamol tablets are prescribed as 1 g t.i.d. for 3 days. How many 500 mg tablets should be dispensed?	Amount to be administered per dose = 1g = 1000 mg Amount to be administered daily (1 g t.i.d) = 1000mg x 3 = 3000 mg Amount to be administered in three days = 3000 mg per day x 3 days = 9000 mg Each tablet is 500 mg. Therefore, in order to supply 9000 mg, the number of tablets needed = $\frac{Total\ amount\ needed}{amount\ in\ each\ tablet} = \frac{9000}{500} = 18\ tablets.\ Answer.$

Q109. What volume in mL of azithromycin Suspension containing 250 mg per 5 mL would provide 500mg per day for three days?	5 mL contain 250 mg. In order to supply the dose of 500 mg, we need 10 mL of the suspension for three days. $$Total\ amount = number\ of\ doses \times size\ of\ dose$$ Total volume of suspension therefore = 3 x 10 = 30 mL. Answer.	
Q110. Calculate the amount of Potassium thiocyanate solution (in mL) that would provide 100 mg of potassium thiocyanate three times a day for 10 days. [Potassium thiocyanate solution contains 2.5 g per 100 mL solution]	Amount needed per day = 100mg x 3 Amount needed in 10 days = 100mg x 3 x 10 = 3000 mg (or 3g) Potassium thiocyanate solution is available as 2.5g per 100 mL. By ratio: $\frac{2.5\ g}{100\ mL} = \frac{3\ g}{x\ mL}$ x = 120 mL. Answer.	

8.1.5 To Calculate the number of doses, total volume to be supplied to the patient for the dosage regimen expressed in a prescription:

Q111. How much of the medicine should be supplied in the following prescriptions?

prescription	Interpretation	Number of doses	Total volume to be supplied
a) 15 mL od x 1/52	15 mL of the medicine to be taken once per day for one week.	1x 3 times a day x 7 days = 21 doses	15 mL x 3 x 7 15 x 21doses = 315 mL
b) 10 mL bd 5/7	10 mL of medicine to be taken 12 hourly for 5 days	1 x 2 times a day x 5 days = 10 doses	10 mL x 10 doses = 100 mL
c) 5 mL qds 1/30	5 mL of medicine to be taken 6 hourly (four times a day) for 1 month.	1 x 4 times per day x 30 days = 120 doses	5 mL x 120 doses = 600mLAnswer.
d) 2.5 mL tds for 10/7	2.5 mL 8 hourly (three times a day) for ten days.	1 x 3 x 10 = 30	2.5 x 30 doses = 75 mL Answer.
e) 200 mLs of a medicine are supplied and instructed to be taken 1 tsp t.i.d. How many days shall the medicine last?	Take 1 teaspoonful (or 5 mL) every 8 hours (= three times a day)	5 x 3 = 15 mL per day	The patient takes 5 mL three time a day = 15 mL per day. For 200 mL, it will supply enough medicine for $\frac{(200\ mL)}{15\ ml/day}$ = 13 days Ans.

How many tablets should be supplied in these prescriptions?

prescription	Interpretation	Number of doses	Total number of tablets to be supplied
Q112. a) Prednisolone tabs 10 mg stat, then 5 mg day 2-5, then 2.5 mg for 5 days. (Each tablet contains 5 mg)	Take prednisolone tablets 10 mg immediately, then 5 mg daily for the next four days, then 2.5 mg for the next 5 days (in total 10 days)	Ten doses in 10 days	Each tablet is 5 mg. day 1 = 2 tablets (10 mg), day 2 -5 = 1 tab/day (4 days) = 4 tablet, day 6-10 = ½ tab (2.5 mg) = 2.5 tabs (supply 3 tablets) Total = 9 tablets
b) ii tab bd 2/52	Take 2 tablets 12 hourly for two weeks	1 dose x 2 times a day x 14 days	1x2x14=28 tablets Answer
c) i tab q6h 7/7	Take 1 tablet every six hours for 7 days	1 x 4 times a day x 7 days	1 x 4 x 7 = 28 tablets. Answer.

Q 113. What volume of liquid (solution, suspension, elixir or emulsion) shall provide the prescribed dose?

prescription	Available concentration	Volume of liquid required to be administered
a) 200 mg b.d.	250mg/ 5mL	$\frac{200}{250} \times 5ml = 4\ mL$ Every 12 hrs. Answer
b) 0.05 mg t.i.d	250 µg /5 mL	$0.05\ mg = 50 \mu g$ $\frac{50}{250} \times 5 = 1\ ml$ every 8 hours
c) 750 mg od	600 mg / 5 mL	$\frac{750}{600} \times 5 = 6.25\ mL$ daily. Ans.
d) 750 mg od	600 mg/mL	$\frac{750}{600} \times 1 = 1.25\ mL$ daily Ans
e) 300 mg od x 5/7	150mg/5 mL	Volume to be dispensed $\frac{300}{150} \times 5 \times 5 days = 50\ mL$ Answer.
f) 114 mg tds x 1/52	228 mL/5 mL	$\frac{114}{228} \times 5ml \times 3\ times\ a\ day \times 7 days$ $= 52.5\ mL$ Supply 55-60 mL to allow for loss during administration
g) 25,000 units for injection	75,000 units/mL	$\frac{25,000}{75,000} \times 1ml = 0.33 mL$
h) 500 µg	1 mg/mL	$1000\ \mu g = 1\ mg$ Thus $500\ \mu g = 0.5\ mg$ Amount required $= \frac{500}{1000} \times 1mL = \frac{1}{2} mL$

8.1.6 To calculate the quantity of an ingredient in a given dose of medicine, when the total amount is known

$$Quantity\ in\ each\ dose = \frac{Quantity\ in\ total\ amount}{Number\ of\ doses}$$

Q114. 62 ½ g of paracetamol powder was used to prepare 250 tablets of paracetamol. How many mgs are represented in each tablet?	$Quantity\ in\ each\ dose = \frac{Quantity\ in\ total\ amount}{Number\ of\ doses}$ Quantity of total amount = 62 ½ g = 62500 mg Number of doses = number of tablets = 250 $Quantity\ in\ each\ tablet = \frac{62500\ mg}{250\ tablets} = 250\ mg\ per\ tablet.$
Q115. Amobarbital elixir contains 440 mg per 100 mL. How many mgs of amobarbital are contained in a teaspoonful dose?	Teaspoon = 5 mL By ratio $\frac{440\ mg}{x\ mg} = \frac{100mL}{5\ mL}$ $x = 22\ mg$ Answer.
Q116. Sodium Fluoride solution for prevention of dental carries was prepared in a concentration of 55mg per 10 mL. The dose of the solution is 10 drops. Calculate the amount of sodium fluoride in each dose [the dispensing dropper is 25 drops per mL)	In each mL there are 25 drops. Therefore, in 10 mL there will be 250 drops. By ratio, $\frac{55mg}{x} = \frac{250\ drops}{10\ drops}$ $x = 2.2\ mg$ Answer.
Q117. Amodiaquine suspension contains 50mg base per 5 mL. a) Calculate the amount of amodiaquine needed to prepare a three-day dose of the suspension. (the dose of a 5-year-old child is 20mL day 1, 20 mL day 2 and 10mL day three). b) How much amodiaquine (in mg) does the child take?	Total volume of the suspension needed = 20 mL + 20 mL + 10 mL = 50 mL Each 5 mL of suspension contains 50 mg of amodiaquine base. a) In order to prepare 50 mL, 500 mg shall be needed b) The child will take 500 mg of amodiaquine base. Answer.

8.1.7 Calculation of drug dose based on Body Weight.

Q118. The dose of praziquantel for treatment of schistosomiasis is 20 mg per kg three times in day. Praziquantel is available as 600 mg tablets. How many tablets should be dispensed to a patient weighing 72 kg?	The dose is 20 mg/ kg three times a day = 20 mg x 3 = 60 mg/kg. The patient's weight is 72 kg. The dose therefore is mg/kg x kg = 60 x 72 = 4320 mg Praziquantel tablets are 600 mg each. Thus the total number of tablets required = $\frac{4320}{600}$ = 7.2 tablets. 8 tablets should be dispensed. For each dose of 20 mg /kg, the patient needs 20 x 72 mg = 1440 mg. These are equivalent to 1440/600 = 2.4 tablets. Practically the patient will be asked to take 2 ½ tablets 8 hourly!!

8.1.9 Calculation of pediatric doses (doses for children)

There is a common saying that a child is not a "small adult". The children's metabolic organs (liver and kidneys) are not fully developed and therefore cannot handle medicines as an adult does. Furthermore, newborn infants are more sensitive to some medicines. In the past, age was considered as enough basis for calculation of children's' dose. But it was later realized that age alone could not be the basis for this purpose. Thus a more dependable criterion would be the child's weight and body surface are which may correlate well with the child body's ability to handle medicines.

The dose is usually expresses as Milligram per kilogram body weight or simply mg/kg body wt.

Formulae for Calculation of Children Doses according to Age:	
1. Young's Rule $\frac{Age\ in\ years}{Age+12}$ =Dose for child	e.g. A child 6 yrs. old: $\frac{6}{6+12}$ = $\frac{1}{3}$ of adult dose
2. Drilling's Rule $\frac{Age\ in\ Years}{20}$ Proportion of adult dose	e.g. A child of 6 years: $\frac{6}{20}$ = $\frac{3}{10}$ of adult dose (=$\frac{1}{3.3}$ adult dose)
3. Cowling's Rule Child's dose = $$\frac{Age\ at\ next\ birthday\ (years) \times Adult\ dose}{24}$$	e.g. next birthday a child will be 7 years old. His dose is $\frac{7\ x\ adult\ dose}{24}$ = $\frac{1}{3.5}$ of adult dose

3. Fried's Rule: $$\text{Dose for an infant} = \frac{Age(in\ Months) x (adult\ dose)}{150}$$	e.g. A child is 6 months old. His dose is $$\frac{(6 x Adult\ dose)}{150} = \frac{1}{25} Adult\ dose$$
4. Clark's Rule: $$\frac{weight\ (in\ lb) x\ (Adult\ dose)}{150(average\ weight\ of\ adult\ in\ lb)} = Dose\ for\ child$$	A child weighs 20 kg. Calculate the fraction of adult dose that a child will be administered with. 1 kg = 2.2 lb., therefore 20 kg = 44 lb. The dose of the child will be $$\frac{22\ x\ Adult\ dose}{150} = \frac{11}{75} adult\ dose$$ (approx. .1/7 fraction).
Q119. The dose of Gentamycin injection is 1.7 mg /k bd wt. How many mL of an injection containing 40 mg/mL should be injected to 85 kg person?	Dose needed = 1.7 mg/kg x 85 kg (weight of patient) =144.5 mg But the vial is 40 mg/mL By proportion: $\frac{1\ mL}{x\ mL} = \frac{40\ mg}{144.5\ mg}$ x = 3.6 mL Answer.
5. When the dose is given as mg /kg body weight, simply multiply the figure with the body weight	
Q120. The daily dose of Chloramphenicol for a child is 25-50 mg per kg body weight in divided doses. Suppose chloramphenicol was prescribed as 10mg/kg bd wt. t.i.d, what dose would a 30kg child get daily?	10 mg t.i.d = 10 mg x 3 daily. For a 30 kg child, the daily dose is: 10 mg/kg x 3 x 30 kg = 900 mg. Answer.
Q121. The adult dose of a drug is 250 mg twice daily (12 hrly). What is the dose for a 3-year-old child/	Child's dose approx. $= \frac{age\ yrs}{age\ yrs+ 12}$ x adult dose $= \frac{3}{3+12}$ x adult dose. $= \frac{3}{15}$ x 250 = 50 mg two times a day
Q122. What is the dose for an 8-month infant if the average dose of an adult is 100mg?	The age is in months. Therefore, use Fried's rule: $$Dose\ of\ infant = \frac{Age(in\ Months) x (adult\ dose)}{150}$$ $\frac{8}{150}$ x 100 = 5.33 mg

Q123. What is the dose of child weighing 45 lb. if the dose of an adult is 250 mg?	You Have been given weight in pounds. Therefore, use Clark's rule: Infant's dose = $\frac{weight\ (in\ lb) \times (Adult\ dose)}{150 (average\ weight\ of\ adult\ in\ lb)}$ $= \frac{45 \times 250}{150} = 75\ mg.\ Answer.$

8.1.10 Calculation of children doses based on body surface area as related to weight.

Doses for children based on age and body weight were found not to be entirely satisfactory. A method was devised to include the surface area of the body. This was considered because the dose depends on metabolic rate, lean body mass and extracellular fluid volume, all being factors which relate to surface area than to age or height. An average adult has a surface area of 1.73 square meters (m²). Approximate doses of children may be obtained by multiplying the adult dose and the ratio

$$\frac{surface\ are\ of\ a\ child\ in\ reation\ to\ his\ weight}{(average\ surface\ area\ of\ the\ adult\ person (1.73\ m^2))}$$

A table showing the relationship of surface are and individual's weight has been designated by several authors. The following table is a combination of tables adapted from Stocklosa M and Ansel H, Pharmaceutical Calculations, and Cooper and Gunn's Dispensing for Pharmaceutical Students.:

Table 4. Relationship between weight and body surface area

Weight in pounds (lb)	Weight in Kg	Square area (m²)	Average corresponding age	Percentage of adult dose
4.4	2	0.15	1-month premature baby	9
5.5	2.5			10
6.6	3	0.20		11.5
7	3.2		At birth	12.5
8.8	4	0.25		14
10	4.5		2months	15
11	5	0.29		16.5
13.2	6	0.33		19
14	6.5		4 months	20
15.4	7	0.37		21
17.6	8	0.40		23
19.8	9	0.43		25
22	10	0.46	12 months (1 year)	25-27
25	11		18 months	30

33	15	0.63	3 years	33-36
40	18		5 years	40
44	20	0.83		48
50	23		7 years	50
55	25	0.95		55
66	30	1.08	10 years	60-62
77	35	1.20		69
80	36		11 years	70
88	40	1.3	12 years	75
99-100	45	1.4	14 years	80-81
121	55	1.58	16 years	90-91
145	65	1.7	20 years	100

The shaded rows simplify the table such that the age (in years) can be related to percent of adult dose as follows:

Age in years: 1   3   7   12

Percent of adult dose   25%   33%   50%   75%

For example, Ciprofloxacin can be given in the dose of 250-750 mg twice daily for five days for treatment of respiratory tract infections. The pediatric dose range can be estimated as follows:

Range	Percent of dose	mg
Adult	**100**	**250-750**
12 yr.	75	177.5-562.5
7 yr.	50	125-375
3 yr.	33	82.5 – 247.5
1 yr.	25	62.5 – 187.5

8.1.11 To determine the dose of a child using body surface area as related to weight and height.

A more precise dose can be calculated combining weight, body surface area (BSA) and height, because height is another factor that influences the body surface. A nomogram that includes all these factors has been designed whereby height and weight have been related to BSA. In order to determine the dose, you have to find out the BSA, by connecting a line interconnecting the weight and the corresponding height of the patient and the third point of the line simply gives the BSA.

Fig 2, A NOMOGRAM FOR ESTIMATING BODY SURFACE ARE BY RELATING HEIGHT AND WEIGHT

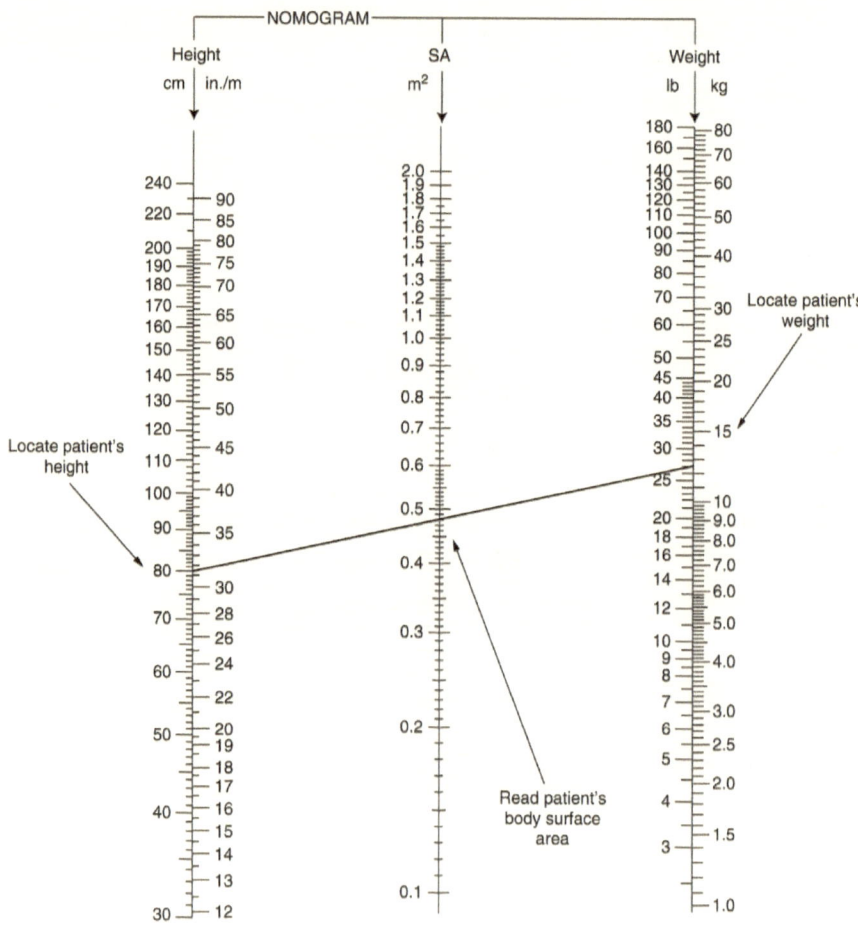

After the BSA has been obtained from the nomogram, the child dose is calculated as follows:

$$\text{Approximate dose of a child} = \frac{BSA \text{ of a child } m^2}{1.73 \ m^2} \times \text{Adult dose}$$

A dose may also be expressed as mg per square meter. Simply multiply the dose in mg/m^2 and the BSA of the child in m^2.

Q124. Using the nomogram above, find the BSA of a child having a height 100 cm and weighing 15 kg.	*Interconnect a line between weight 15kg and height 100 cm. the intercept on the BSA scale shows the BSA as 0.64m^2*
Q125. The daily adult dose of a drug is 10mg. what would be the dose of a child, 110 cm tall weighing 20 kg	*From the nomogram, the BSA of a child weighing 20 kg and height 110 is 0.75m^2* The dose of a child = $\dfrac{BSA\ of\ a\ child\ m^2}{1.73\ m^2}$ x Adult dose $= \dfrac{0.75}{1.73} x10mg = 4.3\ mg\ (approx.\ 4.5\ mg)$
Q126. The dose of a drug is 10mg per m^2. Calculate the dose of a child with BSA 1.45m^2.	The dose = BSA of child x the dose per m^2 The dose = 1.45 m^2 x 10mg/m^2 = 14.5 mg
Q127. The average dose of a drug for an adult is 75 mg. What is the dose for a child who has a body surface area equal to 0.60 m^2?	The child's dose $= \dfrac{surface\ are\ of\ a\ child\ in\ relation\ to\ his\ weight}{(average\ surface\ area\ of\ the\ adult\ person (1.73\ m^2))}$ $\dfrac{0.60}{1.73} x75\ mg = 26\ mg.\ Answer.$
Q128. What is the dose of an average adult if the dose of a drug is 45mg/m^2	The average adult has a body surface are 1.73. therefore, his dose = 45 mg/m^2 x 1.73 = 77.85 mg. Answer
Q129. 180 mL of a cough syrup were prescribed to be taken in four days in a divided dose of three times per day. How many tablespoonfuls should be taken at each dose?	Let the amount (in mL) to be taken at each dose be x. The number of doses = 3 times x 4 days = 12 The mL in of each dose = $\dfrac{total\ volume\ of\ syrup}{total\ numbe\ of\ doses}$ $= \dfrac{180}{12} = 30mL1\ tbsp$ = 15 mL, 30mL= 2 tablespoonfuls
Q130. Calculate the volume of digoxin elixir (50µg/mL) required for provide 1 mg of digoxin for rapid digitalization.	1 mg = 1000 µg There are 50 µg per mL$\dfrac{1\ mL}{x\ mL} = \dfrac{50µg}{1000µg}$ x =20 mL Answer
Q131. Kanamycin injection is administered at the dose of 7.5mg/kg body wt. The injection contains 250mg per mL. How many mL should be	The total dose required = dose (mg/kg) x body weight(kg)

administered to a patient weighing 90 kg?	$= 7.5 \times 90 = 675$ mg But 1 mL contains 250 mg. The number of mL containing 675 can be found by ratio: $\frac{1\,mL}{x\,mL} = \frac{250\,mg}{675\,mg}$ $x = 2.7$ mL
Q132. A bottle contains 100 units of a drug per mL. a) How many mL must a patient take so as to get 80-unit dose? b) If the dose of this drug is 75 units daily, how many days' supply can be obtained from a bottle containing 15 mL of this drug?	a) By ratio, $\frac{1\,mL}{x\,mL} = \frac{100\,units}{80\,units}$ $x = \frac{1 \times 80}{100} = 0.8\,mL$ Answer. b) If 1 mL has 100 units, 15 mL shall have 15×100 units $= 1500$ units. And if the daily dose = 75 units, then 1500 units shall supply $\frac{1500}{75}$ doses or dose for 20 days. Answer.
Q133. A prescription orders 10 units to be administered three times a day for five days. The medicine to be supplied is in a solution as 15units per 5 mL. How many mL of this medicine will you supply?	Total number of units to be administered in five days = 10 units x 3 times a day x 5 days = 150 units The medicine is available as 15 units/mL. By ratio $\frac{1\,mL}{x\,mL} = \frac{15\,units}{150\,units}$ $x = 1\,ml \times \frac{150\,units}{15\,units} = 10\,mL$ Answer.
Q134. The pediatric dose of Nelfinavir is 25-30 mg /kg three times daily. Calculate the amount to be given for each single dose for a child weighing 33 pounds	First of all, convert the weight pounds to kg. 1 lb = 2.2 kg 33lb = 33/2.2 =15 kg. The daily dose for a 15kg child = $15 \times (25\text{-}30)$ mg $= 375\text{-}450$ mg per day But the dose is divided into three administrations per day Thus the child is given $(375 - 450) \div 3$ $= 125\text{-}150$ mg three time a day or 8 hourly. Answer.
Q135. Digoxin, a medicine for treating heart failure is to be administered to a premature infant with a birth weight 1.2 kg. The dose of digoxin in premature infant has been estimated at 20µg/kg in three unequally divided doses of ½, ¼, and ¼. How much digoxin should be administered in this infant?	The dose = µg/kg x kg = 20µg/kg x 1.2 kg = 24µg This dose should be subdivided in ½, ¼, and ¼ Thus the dose should be given as 12µg, 6µg and 6µg

CHAPTER 9

EXPRESSION OF CONCENTRATIONS IN PHARMACEUTICAL PREPARATIONS

9.1 Introduction

The concentration of liquid medicines may be expression in various ways. The most common ones are "percentage" strength (%) and "Ratio" strength. The concentration may be weight-in-weight (w/w), weight-in-volume (w/v) or volume-in-volume (v/v). Sometimes in biochemistry, concentration is expressed as mg%. Concentration of very dilute solutions is expressed as "parts per million" or ppm. Other forms in which concentration may be expressed include milliequivalents per liter (mEq/L), millimoles per liter (mMol/L), Normality, Molality and Molarity.

9.2 Percent.

Percent is a phenomenon encountered very frequently in pharmacy. It is used in expressing a concentration of a solution or a mixture, amount of a drug available to the body in relation to the administered dose, part of a drug metabolized or which reaches the desired site in the body, profit or loss of sales and so forth. The term **percent** expressed as %, means "per hundred", "in a hundred" or "by hundred".

20% means 20 parts in a total of 100 parts, which also means $\frac{20}{100}$ or 0.2

$$5\% = \frac{5}{100} = 0.05 \qquad = 50\% = \frac{50}{100} = \frac{1}{2} \qquad 12.5\% = \frac{12.5}{100} = \frac{1}{8}$$

Percent is a ratio of a given value to 100 and therefore percent has no units.

Q136. What is 10% of 8000 tablets?	Multiply the percent (the ratio of the value to 100) by the number of tablets $= \frac{10}{100} \times 8000 = 800$
Q137. In a batch of 900,000 tablets, 650 tablets were defective. What is the percentage of defective tablets in this batch?	$\frac{650}{900,000} = \frac{X}{100}$ $X = 0.072\%$ Answer.
The percent can be changed to a fraction or expressed as a decimal. To change the percent to a fraction, the percent number becomes the numerator and 100 is the denominator.	
Q138. change 26%, 0.075%, 12.5% and 50% to fractions.	$26\% = \frac{26}{100} = \frac{13}{50}$ $0.075\% = \frac{0.075}{100} = \frac{0.015}{50} = \frac{0.03}{10}$

| | $12.5\% = \frac{12.5}{100} = \frac{1}{8}$ |
| | $50\% = \frac{50}{100} = \frac{1}{2}$ |

To change a fraction to a percent, put the fraction in form having 100 as a denominator, multiply by 100 so that the numerator becomes the percent. For instance, in order to convert 1/8 to percent, express the fraction as follows

$\frac{1}{8} = \frac{X}{100}$ $X = \frac{100}{8} = 12.5$ Therefore $\frac{1}{8} = \frac{12.5}{100} = 12.5\%$

To convert $\frac{35}{90}$ to percent: $\frac{35}{90} = \frac{X}{100}$, $X = \frac{100 \times 35}{90} = \frac{38.9}{100} = 38.9\%$

Q 139. Change the following fractions to percentages: $\frac{1}{5}, \frac{3}{8}, \frac{1}{2}, \frac{4}{9}$, and ¾	$\frac{1}{5} = \frac{20}{100} = 20\%$
	$\frac{3}{8} = \frac{37.5}{100} = 37.5\%$
	$\frac{1}{2} = \frac{50}{100} = 50\%$
	$\frac{4}{9} = \frac{44.44}{100} = 44.44\%$
	$\frac{3}{4} = \frac{75}{100} = 75\%$

In order to make it easy during computations or calculations, it is convenient to change percentage to decimals. In order to do this, drop the % sign and divide the expressed numerator by 100

Thus $10\% = \frac{10}{100} = 0.1$ $13\% = \frac{13}{100} = 0.13$ $0.075\% = \frac{0.075}{100} = 0.00075$

Q140. Express 45%, 0.12%, 99% and 0.004% as decimals	$45\% = \frac{45}{100} = 0.45$
	$0.12\% = \frac{0.12}{100} = 0.0012$
	$99\% = \frac{99}{100} = 0.99$
	$0.004\% = \frac{0.004}{100} = 0.00004 = 4 \times 10^{-5}$

9.3 Expression of liquid concentrations

Pharmaceutical liquid preparations such as solutions, mixtures, lotions, syrups, elixirs, suspensions and emulsions, have their concentrations expressed as parts per 100 parts. For example, you may have 20g of a substance in 100 mL of the solution or 100 g of the solution. For solutions of liquid –in-liquid, the concentration is expressed as the volume of on liquid to 100 mL of the solution.

Concentrations of weak solutions are frequently expressed as a ratio of 1 part to a number of similar parts, e.g. one part in 1000 parts, expressed as 1:1000. The difference of this expression from percentage is that whereas percentages are expressed as number of parts per 100 parts, ratio strength expresses one part of a substance in several parts of the mixture. Thus 5% means 5 part in 100 parts (or 5:100), but when expressed as ratio strength 5 % will be expressed as 1:20 which means one part per 20 parts.

The concentration is thus expressed as

1. *Percent weight-in- volume* (%w/v) which means the number of grams(g) of a constituent or ingredient in 100 mL of the liquid preparation whether it is a solution, mixture or otherwise (NOT 100 mL OF THE SOLVENT!)

> *For example, 0.9% sodium chloride solution means there is 0.9 g of sodium chloride in 100 mL of the solution*

2. *Percent weight-in-weight* (%w/w). which means the number of grams (g) of the constituent in 100 g of the of the liquid preparation (NOT 100 mL OF THE SOLVENT).

> *For example, 3% (w/w) coal tar ointment means that we have 3 g of coal tar in 100 g of the ointment.*

3. *Percent volume –in-volume (% v/v)* which means the number of mL of a constituent in 100 mL of the solution (NOT 100 mL OF THE SOLVENT)

> *For example, Pediatric codeine linctus is said to be 20% v/v. This means it contains 20 mL of codeine linctus in 100mL*

When % is not qualified, i.e. without w/v, w/w or v/v, then if the preparation in question is a solid or semi solid, we assume that the concentration is w/w. For liquid preparations containing solid solutes, we assume that the concentration is w/v. For solution of liquids–in-liquids, unqualified concentration is assumed to be v/v. For solutions of gases in liquids (e.g. carbon dioxide in water), % w/v is assumed.

4. *Ratio strength* Whereby the concentration is expressed as one part per several parts of the mixture.

9.4 EXPRESSION OF CONCENTRATION AS "PERCENT STRENGTH"

If you are asked to prepare a pharmaceutical preparation given the percent concentration of the ingredients required, it is easy to compute how much of each ingredient is required for any given volume of the preparation required.

Q141. How much iodine is contained in 500 mL Lugol's solution? (in the monographs, Lugol's solution contains 5% w/v iodine). *(The question is the same as "how much iodine is required to prepare 500 mL of Lugol's solution?)*	5% w/v means 5 g in 100 mL solution. If 5g are in 100 mL, how much iodine is in 500 mL? $$\frac{5g}{100mL} = \frac{Xg}{500\ mL}$$ $X = \frac{500 \times 5}{100} = 25g$ Answer.
Q142. ℞ Podophyllum resin 25% Cpd Benzoin tincture ad 50 mL How much podophyllum is required to make the preparation above?	The preparation is 25%, which means 25 g in 100 mL solution. We are asked to prepare 50 mL. therefore $\frac{25}{100} = \frac{X}{50}$ $X = \frac{50 \times 25}{100} = 12.5\ g$
Q143. Calculate the amount of ingredients required to prepare 5 L of a 0.2% solution of a substance?	0.2% means 0.2 g of the substance in 100 g of solution. Thus if 0.2 g is in 100 mL, how much will be contained in 5L or 5000 mL? $$\frac{0.2\ g}{100\ mL} = \frac{X\ g}{5000\ mL}$$ $X = \frac{5000 \times 0.2}{100} = 10\ g$
Q144. There are 15g of a substance in 75 mL of a solution. Express this concentration in % strength w/v	There are 15 g are in 75 mL. In order to find the percent strength, we need to find out how many g are contained in 100 mL $$\frac{15\ g}{x\ g} = \frac{75\ mL}{100\ mL}$$ $X = \frac{15 \times 100}{75} = 20$ The strength is 20% w/v Answer.
Q145. Pentobarbital injection is prepared as 50mg/mL solution. Express this concentration as % strength	To find the percent strength we need to calculate the amount of the ingredient in 100 mL If 50 mg are in 1mL how many g are in 100 mL? First of all, convert 50 mg to g We know that 1000mg = 1g, therefore 50 mg = 0.05g By ratio, $\frac{0.05g}{X\ g} = \frac{1\ mL}{100mL}$ $X = \frac{100 \times 0.05}{1} = 5$

	$\frac{5}{100} = 5\%w/v$ Answer
Q146. 425 g of sucrose are dissolved in enough water to make ½ liter solution. Calculate the percent strength of the solution	There are 425g in ½ liter. We know that 1 liter = 1000 mL, therefore ½ liter = 500 mL To find the percentage, find how many g are in 100 mL $\frac{425\,g}{X\,g} = \frac{500\,mL}{100\,mL}$ $X = 85.$ Thus $\frac{85}{100} = 85\%$ Ans.
Q147. How many mL of iodine tincture (2% w/v) can be made from 125 g of iodine?	2% means that there are 2g in 100 mL. how many mL shall hold 125 g? $\frac{2\,g}{125\,g} = \frac{100\,mL}{X\,mL}$ $X = 6250\,mL$ Answer.
Q148. How many liters of Normal Saline (0.9% w/v sodium chloride) can be made if you are provided with 2.4 kg sodium chloride?	0.9% w/v means 0.9 g in 100 mL. We know that 1kg = 1000 g. Hence 2.4 kg = 2400 g Therefore $\frac{0.9\,g}{2400\,g} = \frac{100\,mL}{X\,mL}$ $X = 266666.67\,mL$ But 1000 mL = 1 L. therefore, 266666.67mL = **26.67L**
Q149. Liquefied phenol is used in the concentration of 2.5%v/v as a preservative in Calamine lotion. How much liquid phenol is needed to prepare ¼ liter of Calamine lotion?	2.5% v/v means 2.5 mL in 100 mL of solution. We know that 1 liter = 1000mL. therefore, ¼ liter = 250 mL If 2.5 mL are in 100 mL, how many mL are in 250 mL? $\frac{2.5\,mL}{X\,mL} = \frac{100\,mL}{250\,mL}$ $X = \frac{250 \times 2.5}{100} = 6.25\,mL$ Answer. **This problem can also be solved by using the following formula:** mL of active ingredient (AI) = Volume in mL X Percentage (in decimal expression): we know that $2.5\% = \frac{2.5}{100}$ Therefore, mL of phenol required = $250\,mL \times \frac{2.5}{100}$ $= 250 \times 0.025 = 6.25\,mL$
Q150. How many mL of resorcinol should be used to prepare 450 mL of 15% v/v lotion?	mL of active ingredient = Volume of preparation X percent of active ingredient $= 450\,mL \times \frac{15}{100} = 450 \times 0.15 = 67.5\,mL$ This can also be done by proportions: $\frac{15}{X} = \frac{100}{450}$ $X = \frac{450 \times 15}{100} = 67.5\,mL$

Q151. A sunscreen lotion contains 5% v/v methyl salicylate. Calculate the number of mLs required to prepare 2 liters of the lotion	Active ingredient (AI) (mL) = Volume of lotion (mL) x % AI. $$= 2L \times \frac{5}{100}$$ $$= 2000\ mL \times \frac{5}{100} = 100\ mL$$
Q152. How many grams of sucrose are required to make 250 mL of 65% w/v solution?	Weight of solute (in g) = (Weight of solution in g) X (%) expresses as decimal) $$= 250 \times \frac{65}{100} = 162.5\ g$$
DIFFERENTIATE w/v FROM v/v Q153. How many grams of sucrose must be dissolved in 250 mL of water to make a 65% **w/w** solution?	Percent weight-in-weight indicates the number of parts by weight of active ingredient that are contained in the total weight of the solution or mixture (which is considered as 100 parts by weight. For a 65 % solution, it means the active ingredient is 65% by weight, and water is 35% by weight. 250mL of water weigh 250 g and contributes 35% by weight. Let us find the number of g of sucrose that should be dissolved in this amount of water to make a 65% w/w solution: $\frac{65\%}{35\%} = \frac{X\ g}{250\ g}$ X = 464.3 g Answer.
Q154. How many grams of a substance should be dissolved in 1.8L of water to make a 15 % w/w solution?	If the active ingredient is 15% by weight, water should be 100% -15% = 85% by weight 1.8 L of water = 1800mL of water, which weighs 1800 g $\frac{85\ (\%)}{15\ (\%)} = \frac{1800\ (g)}{X\ (g)}$ $X = \frac{15 \times 1800}{85} = 317.65\ g$ *This problem can also be done as follows:* Let the amount of the substance required be X g Then the total weight of the substance and water $= X + 1800\ g$ If the concentration is 15%, it means that $\frac{X}{X + 1800} \times 100 = 15\%$ 15(X+1800) =100X 15X + 27,000 = 100X 27,000 = 85 X [subtract 15X from both sides] X = 317.65 g

Q155. How many grams of tannic acid must be dissolved in 480 mL of Glycerin to make a 12% w/w solution? (Glycerin has specific gravity of 1.25)	Weight = volume X Specific gravity 480 mL of glycerin weigh 480 x 1.25 = 600 g **Method 1:** If the solution is 12%w/w, then tannic acid is 12% and glycerin is 88%. The weight of tannic acid can be found by proportion: $\frac{12}{88} = \frac{X}{600}$ X = 81.81 g Answer. **Method 2:.** Weight of glycerin = 600g Let the weight of tannic acid be T. this weight contributes 12%. Therefore $\frac{T}{T+600} = \frac{12}{100}$ $100T = 12T + 7200$ $88T = 7200$ T = 81.81 g Answer
Q156. What is the concentration w/w of a syrup containing 850 g of sucrose in 1 liter of syrup? (the specific gravity of the syrup is 1.3)	First of all, find the weight of the syrup. Weight of 1 liter of syrup = volume (mL) x Specific gravity = 1000 mL x 1.3 = 1300g Concentration w/w = $\frac{850\ g\ (wt\ of\ sucrose)}{1300\ g\ (weight\ of\ syrup)}$ x 100 = 65.38% w/w Answer. OR by using proportions, $\frac{850}{1300} = \frac{X}{100}$ X = 65.38% w/w
Q157. Calculate the percent (weight-in-weight) of a solution made by dissolving 19.8 g potassium chloride in 66 mL water.	66 mL weigh 66 g. Total weight = 66 g + 19.8 g = 85.8 g. If the weight of potassium chloride is 19.8, then concentration w/w = $\frac{19.8}{85.8}$ x 100 = 20.1% w/w
Q158. How many grams of hydrocortisone are required to make 15 g of a topical cream containing 2% (w/w) hydrocortisone,	The concentration 2% w/w means that there are 2 g hydrocortisone in 100 g ointment. We need to calculate how many g of hydrocortisone will be in 15 g of ointment: $\frac{2}{100} = \frac{X}{15}$ X = 0.3 g Answer.
Q159. Calculate the amount of Procaine hydrochloride required to prepare 150 suppositories each weighing 1.5 g and containing 0.25% w/w procaine hydrochloride.	Total weight of suppositories = 150 suppositories x 1.5 g = 225 g If the suppositories contain 0.25%w/w, it means there is 0.25 g procaine HCl for every 100 g. We are required to calculate how many grams are in 225g.

	$\frac{0.25}{100} = \frac{X}{225}$ $x = 0.5625\ g\ (562.5\ mg)$
Q160. ℞. Tragacanth, finely powdered 22.5g Acacia finely powdered 30 g Starch, finely powdered 30 g Sucrose, finely powdered 67.5 g Calculate the percentage of each ingredient w/w	Total weight = 22.5+30+30+67.5=150g $Tragacanth = \frac{22.5}{150} \times 100 = 15\%w/w$ $Acacia = \frac{30}{150} \times 100 = 20\%w/w$ $Starch = \frac{30}{150} \times 100 = 20\ \%w/w$ $Sucrose = \frac{67.5}{150} \times 100 = 45\%w/w$

Q161. A pharmacist is asked to modify Whitfield's ointment using the following formula:
Whitfield's Ointment 90 g
   Salicylic acid   30g
   Yellow paraffin ad 450 g
 	
Whitfield's ointment contains 3% salicylic acid. Calculate the percentage of salicylic acid in the final product
	Whitfield's ointment contains 3 % salicylic acid (w/w). This means that there are 3 g of salicylic acid in 100 g of ointment. Let us find out how many grams of salicylic acid are in 90 g of the ointment:
	$\frac{3}{100} = \frac{X}{90}$ $X = 2.7\ g$
	A further 30 g amount of salicylic acid has been added, which makes the total amount of salicylic acid to be 2.7g+30g = 32.7g
	
	Total weight of the final ointment = 450 g
	Thus the % of salicylic acid in the final ointment =
	$\frac{32.7}{450} \times 100 = 7.27\ \%\ (w/w)$ Answer.
	
	OR $\frac{32.7}{450} = \frac{X}{100}$ $X = 7.27\%\ w/w$

Q162. 10 grams boric acid are dissolved in 150 mL of water. Calculate the concentration w/v and w/w	For w/v concentration we need to know the volume of the solution after adding 10 g boric acid to 150 mL of water. If the amount of boric acid was small (let us say 1 g) then there is no significant change in volume and we can assume a concentration being 1/150 x100 = 0.67% For the w/w concentration we calculate as follows: 150 mL water weigh 150 g. We are adding 10 g boric acid. The final weight is therefore 150 +10 = 160g The concentration w/w = $\frac{10}{160} \times 100 = 6.25\ \%\ (w/w)$ Ans. OR $\frac{10\ g\ Boric\ acid}{160\ g\ weight\ of\ solution} = \frac{X}{100}$ $X=6.25\%\ w/w$

9.5 EXPRESSION OF CONCENTRATION AS RATIO STRENGTH

9.5.1 Ratio strength is used in weak solutions or mixtures (i.e. when a solute is in small concentration).

An expression 1:1000 means that

  i. For solid-in-liquids, there is 1 gram of solute or constituent in 1000 mL of solution or liquid preparation
  ii. For liquids-in-liquids, 1 milliliter of constituent is in 1000 mL of solution or liquid preparation
  iii. For solid in solid, there is 1 gram of constituent in 1000 gram of a mixture of the solids.

Q163. Express the following percentages as ratio strength: a) 0.25%, d) 0.005%, b) 55%, e) 4.5%, c) ½ %, f) 1/25 %	a) 0.25% means $\frac{0.25}{100}$ or 0.25 parts in 100 parts. Ratio strength is expressed as 1 part in several parts. In this case we ask ourselves, if 0.25 parts are in 100 parts, 1 part is in how many parts? $\frac{0.25\,(\%)}{100\,\%} = \frac{1\,part}{X\,parts}$ $X = \frac{100 \times 1}{0.25} = 400$ 0.25% expressed as Ratio strength = 1 : 400, Ans. b) $\frac{55}{100} = \frac{1}{x}$ $x = 1.82$. Ratio strength = 1:1.82 c) ½% = $\frac{0.5}{100} = \frac{1}{x}$ $x = 200$. = 1:200 d) $\frac{0.005}{100} = \frac{1}{x}$ $x = 20{,}000$ = 1: 20,000 e) $\frac{4.5}{100} = \frac{1}{x}$ $x = 22.22$ = 1: 22.22 f) $\frac{1}{25}\% = \frac{0.04}{100} = \frac{1}{x}$ $x = 25$ =1:25
Q164. Express each of the following as ratio strength: a) 0.5 mg of active ingredient in 2 mL of solution b) 2 g of active ingredient in 300 mL solution c) 0.25g in 5mL	a) 0.5 mg = 0.0005g. If 0.0005 g are in 2 mL, 1 g will be in how many mL? $\frac{0.0005\,g}{1\,g} = \frac{2\,mL}{X\,ml}$ $X = 4000$ Ratio strength is = 1:4000 h) $\frac{2\,g}{1\,g} = \frac{300\,mL}{x\,mL}$ $X = 150$ ratio strength = 1:150 c) $\frac{(0.25\,g)}{1\,g} = \frac{5\,mL}{X\,mL}$ $X = 20$ Ratio strength = 1:20

Q165. Express the following ratio strengths as percentages: a) 1:1000 c) 1:80 b) 1:20,000 d) 1: 100,000	a) 1: 1000 means that there is 1 g in 1000 mL liquid Preparation (solution, suspension etc.) or there is 1g of a solid in 1000 g of solid mixture. In order to change this ratio into percent strength we need to find out how many grams shall be in 100 mL or in 100 g of a mixture as the case may be. $\frac{1 \,(g \text{ or } mL)}{X \,(g \text{ or } mL)} = \frac{1000 \,(g \text{ or } mL)}{100 \,(g \text{ or } mL)}$ $X = 0.1$ This means that there is 0.1 g in 100 mL or 0.1 mL in 100 mL or 0.1 g in 100 g. Either case, this means the concentration is = 0.1% Answer. b) $\frac{1}{X} = \frac{20{,}000}{100}$ $X = 0.005$ = 0.005% Answer c) $\frac{1}{X} = \frac{80}{100}$ $X = 1.25$ = 1.25% Answer d) $\frac{1}{X} = \frac{100{,}000}{100}$ $X = 0.001$ = 0.001% Answer. TO CONVERT RATIO STRENGTH TO PERCENT STRENGTH, SIMPLY EXPRESS THE RATIO STRENGTH AS A RECIPROCAL FRACTION AND MULTIPLY IT BY 100: $1:X = \frac{1}{X} \times 100$ e.g 1: 1500 $= \frac{1}{1500} \times 100 = 0.067\%$
To solve **problems involving ratio strength** it is suggested and recommended to translate the ratio strength in the problems to percent strength and then solve them by the rules and methods of percentages discussed earlier.	
Q166. A prescription asks you to prepare ½ liter of 1:5000 potassium permanganate (PP) solution. How many grams of PP do you require?	First convert the concentration 1: 5000 into percent strength, and solve as usual. $1:5000 = \frac{1}{5000} \times 100 = 0.02\%$ ½ liter = 500 mL PP required = $500 \times \frac{0.02}{100} = 0.1$ g Answer Or by proportion: 1:5000 means that there is 1 gram in 5000 mL. to convert to percentage strength, find out how much shall be in 500 mL: $\frac{1}{X} = \frac{5000}{500}$ $X = \frac{500}{5000}$ = 0.1 g Answer.

Q167.
℞ Adrenaline solution 1:1000   10 mL
   Simple syrup   Ad   80 mL
       Sig 1 tsp bd
 	
Calculate the concentration of adrenaline in the preparation and the amount of adrenaline in each dose
	$1:1000 = \frac{1}{1000} \times 100 = 0.1\%$
	
	10 mL of 0.01% adrenaline contains
	
	$\frac{0.01}{100} \times 10 = 0.001\ g$
	
	It is this same amount available in the final volume of 80 mL. So the concentration of adrenaline in the preparation
	
	$= \frac{0.001}{80} \times 100 = 0.00125\%$
	
	OR $\frac{0.001\ g}{X\ g} = \frac{80\ mL}{100\ mL}$ $X = 0.00125\%$
	
	The dose is 1 teaspoonful, equivalent to 5 mL. We are asked to calculate the amount of adrenaline in this amount. If the concentration is 0.00125%, it means that 0.00125 g is in 100 mL. let us calculate the amount in 5 mL:
	
	$\frac{0.00125}{x} = \frac{100}{5}$ $X = 0.0000625\ g$ or $0.0625\ mg$

Q168 ℞Hexachlorophene1:250 Hydrophilic Ointment Ad 15g Sig apply on wound after cleaning with Eusol solution. How many milligrams are required to compound this prescription?	$1:250 = \frac{1}{250} \times 100 = 0.4\%$ 15 grams contain $15 \times \frac{0.4}{100} = 0.06\ g = 60\ mg$ OR If 1 g is in 250 g, how much will be in 15 g? $\frac{1}{X} = \frac{250}{15} =$ $X = 0.06$

9.5.1.1 To convert Percent strength to milligram per milliliter (mg/mL), grams per liter(g/L)

Concentration of Infusions and other solutions expressed as percent strength or ratio strength may be needed to be expressed as milligram per liter or grams per liter. There are simple techniques to perform these conversions.

To convert percent strength to mg /mL, multiply the percent by ten: mg/mL = % x 10 Q169. Express 5% w/v in milligram per milliliter	5 x 10 = 50mg/mLPROOF: 5% w/v = 5 g in 100 mL = 5000 mg in 100 mL = 50 mg in 1 mL = 50mg/mL

	OR $\frac{5000}{X} = \frac{100}{1}$ $X = 50$ $= 50$ mg/mL Answer.
Q170. Change 75% to mg/mL	75 x 10 = 750 mg /mL Answer
Q171 Erythromycin topical solution has 2% w/v strength. Express this concentration in mg/mL	2x10 = 20 mg/mL Answer.
To convert ratio strength to mg/mL, divide the ratio strength by 1000, to get the number of mL containing 1 mg Ratio strength ÷ 1000 = number of mL containing 1 mg Q172. Convert 1:20000 (w/v) to mg/mL	20,000 ÷ 1000 = mg/ 20 mL PROOF: 1:20,000 means that 1 gram is in 20,000 mL, = 1000mg in 20,000 mL. Therefore 1 mg in 20 mL You can easily calculate how many mgs in 1 mL = 0.05 mg/mL
Q173. How many milligrams of isofluorate are contained in 1 mL of a 1:15.000 ophthalmic oily Isofluorate solution?	15,000÷ 1000 = 1 mg in 15mL = 0.067mg/mL
To convert grams per liter (g/L) to milligrams per milliliter (mg/L), convert the numerator to milligrams and divide the number of milliliters in the denominator to obtain mg/mL Q174. A disinfectant is said to have 2 g per liter. Covert this concentration to mg/mL	Covert 2 g into milligrams, and 1 liter into milliliters: 2g = 2000mg. $\frac{2000mg}{1000\ ml} = 2\ mg/L$ PROOF: $\frac{2g}{liter} = \frac{2000mg}{liter} = \frac{2000mg}{1000 mililiters} = 2mg/mL$ 150 g are in 300 mL. We need to find out how many g are in

Q175. A 300 mL preparation is said to have 150 g of active ingredient. Express this concentration in grams/liter, and in mg/mL	$\dfrac{150}{X} = \dfrac{300}{1}\ \dfrac{1\ mL}{}$ $X = 500 = 500\ g/L$ In order to convert to mg/L, Convert 150 g to mg = 150,000 mg Divide the numerator by the number of milliliters = 150,000/300 = 500 mg/mL Answer. $500\ g/L = \dfrac{500g}{1000\ mL} = \dfrac{500000mg}{1000\ mL} = 500 mg/mL$
Q176. Convert 1.5 g in 210 mLs to mg/L	$\dfrac{1500}{210} = 7.14\ mg/mL$ Answer.

9.5.2 Concentration expressed as parts per million (ppm)

Occasionally, and particularly for very dilute solutions, concentration is expressed as parts per million(ppm). Whereas a 10% solution means that there are 10 parts per 100 parts, 10 ppm there is 1 part of solute per 1 million parts of solution. Likewise, 5 ppm means there are 5 parts of solute per 1 million parts of solution. An example of a medicine expressed as ppm in concentration is sodium fluoride, a preservative used to prevent tooth decay. The drug is toxic and is only needed in minute quantities, 3 ppm which means 3 g in 1 million mL of water. Chlorine is used to cleanse the water in swimming pools, but the concentration is so low that it is expressed as ppm

Q177. 300 mg of a certain drug were dissolved in 10 liters. Express this concentration as parts per million (ppm)	Ppm means number of grams of solute in 1000000 parts of solution 300 mg = 0.3 g 10 liters = 10,000 mL 0.3 g is in 10,000 mL. How many grams are in 1000000 mL? $\dfrac{0.3\ g}{X\ g} = \dfrac{10,000\ mL}{1,000,000\ mL}\quad X = 30\ ppm$
Q178. Fluoride water supply is 0.9 ppm. Express this concentration in percent strength, ratio strength and mg/mL.	0.9 ppm means 0.9g per 1,000,000 mL a) To find % strength, calculate the amount in 100 mL $\dfrac{0.9\ g}{X\ g} = \dfrac{1,000,000\ mL}{100\ mL}\quad X = 0.00009\%$ b) to express the concentration as ratio strength, find out the volume that will have 1 g if 0.9 g are in 1 million mL $\dfrac{0.9\ g}{1\ g} = \dfrac{1,000,000\ mL}{X\ mL}\quad X = 1111111.11$ Ratio strength = 1: 1111111 c) To find mg/mL, find the number of mg to be found

	in 1 mL if 0.9 g are in 1000000 mL $$0.9\ g = 900\ mg$$ $$\frac{900}{X} = \frac{1000000}{1} \qquad X = 0.0009\ mg/mL$$ ** *You can use % strength to calculate mg/mL by multiplying the % by 10 as above:* $$Mg/mL = \% \times 10$$ $$= 0.00009 \times 10 = 0.0009\ mg/mL$$
Q179. Two milligrams of gentian violet were added to 1-liter Ethanol in order to color it to avoid misuse. Express this concentration as parts per million	$2\ mg = 0.002\ g$ $$\frac{0.002\ g}{X\ g} = \frac{1{,}000\ mL}{1{,}000{,}000\ mL} \qquad X = 2 \quad = 2\ ppm$$

CHAPTER 10

CALCULATIONS INVOLVING FOMULATIONS: REDUCING AND ENLARGING FORMULAE

10.1. Introduction

One of important tasks of pharmacists, pharmaceutical technicians and pharmaceutical assistants is to compound pharmaceutical preparations. The preparations made in a pharmacy are from proven formulas that have been tested and are listed in Inernational pharmacopoeia such as the United States Pharmacopeia (USP), National Formulary(NF), the British pharmacopoeia (BP) and Martindale the Extra pharmacopoeia. Other countries may also have their own local formularies. These formulae list the amount of each ingredient needed to make a certain amount of the preparation. Official formulae are usually based on 1000 mL or 1000 g products, though sometimes we come across formulae based on 100 mL 0r 100 g. A task may require compounding of smaller or larger quantity than the one stated in the formula. Thus we may need to reduce or expand the formula given. Either case, the ingredients' proportions must remain the same as in the original formula.

$$\frac{Total\ amount\ specified\ in\ the\ formula}{Total\ amount\ desired} = \frac{Quantity\ of\ each\ ingredient\ in\ the\ formula}{Quantity\ of\ each\ ingredient\ in\ the\ amount\ desired}$$

The quantity may be in terms of weight, volume or just parts.

- When the total or final volume or weight of ingredients in the formula is not stated, you must first of all determine the total weight by adding individual weight or volume of ingredients
- Calculate the factor of reduction or expansion of the formulary by dividing the total quantity required by the total quantity stated in the formula
- To reduce the formula in the metric system, divide by the power of 10 by moving the decimal point to the left the required number of places for each ingredient. To enlarge the formula, multiply by a power of 10 by moving the decimal point to the right the required number of places.

Q180. From the following formula, calculate the quantity of each ingredient required to prepare 350 mL of the mixture:	Total quantity stated in the formula = 1000 mL Total quantity required = 350 mL Conversion factor = 350/1000 = 0.35
Paracetamol 24 g Benzoic acid 1 g EDTA 1 g Propylene glycol 150 mL Ethanol (90%) 150 mL Saccharin 1.8 g Water 200 mL Flavor q.s. Sorbital solution, Ad. 1000 mL	All ingredients will be multiplied by the conversion factor to obtain required quantity of each ingredient Thus: Paracetamol = 24 x 0.35 = 8.4 g Benzoic acid = 1 x 0.35 = 0.35 g EDTA = 1 x 0.35 = 0.35 g Propylene glycol = 150 x 0.35 =52.5 g Ethanol = 150 x 0.35 =52.5 g Saccharin = 1.8 x 0.35 =0.63 g Water = 200 x 0.35 = 70 mL Flavor (a small amount which does not affect the final volume significantly. It may be a drop or two) Sorbitol solution, add to make 350 mL

Q181.	Stated amount in the formula = 100 mL
℞ Hexachlorophene 0.1 g Cetyl alcohol 0.5 g Isopropyl alcohol 70 g Purified water Ad 100 mL Calculate the quantity of each ingredient required to prepare 1 liter of the lotion	Required quantity = 1 liter = 1000 mL Conversion factor = $\frac{1000}{100}$ = 10 Multiply each ingredient by 10 (simply shift the decimal point to the right or for whole numbers add a zero. Hexachlorophene = 0.1 x 10 = 1 Cetyl alcohol = 0.5 x 10 = 5 Isopropyl alcohol = 70 x10 = 700 Purified water add enough to make 1000 mL of the lotion
Q182. The formula for pediatric Azithromycin suspension is125 mg/5 mL. We need to prepare 500 bottles each containing 50 mL suspension. How many grams of azithromycin are required?	Total volume of the suspension required = 50 mL x 500 bottles = 25,000 mL The concentration is 125 mg per 5 mL. We need to calculate how many grams are 25,000 mL $\frac{125\ mg}{X\ mg} = \frac{5\ mL}{25,000\ mL}$ X = 625,000 mg = 625 g Ans.
Q183. ℞ Antipyrine 540 mg Benzocaine 110 mg Glycerin 10 mL Sig: Otic solution Supply 5000 bottles. How much of each ingredient is required?	The formula is for 10 mL bottle. 5000 bottles are needed. All ingredients must be multiplied by 5000 Antipyrine: 540 mg x 5000 = 2,700,000 mg= 2.7 kg Benzocaine: 110 x 5000 = 550,000 mg = 0.55 kg Glycerin: 10 mL x 5000 = 50000 mL= 5 L
Q184. An anti-hypertensive syrup has been prescribed to contain hydrochlorthiazide 6.5 mg / 5 mL and captopril 12.5 mg / 5 mL How much of each ingredient is required to supply 5 liters of the syrup? How many bottles of 100 mL will be able to be made from this volume?	We need to calculate how much of each ingredient will be in 5 liters or 5000 mL Hydrochlorthiazide: 6.5 mg are in 5 mL; how much is in 5000 mL? $\frac{6.5}{x} = \frac{5\ mL}{5000\ mL}$ X = 65,000 mg = 65 g Answer Captopril: 12.5 mg are in 5 mL; how many mgs are in 5000 mL? $\frac{12.5}{X} = \frac{5\ mL}{5,000\ mL}$ X = 12,500 mg = 12.5 g Answer. If we have 5 L (or 5000 mL) how many 100 mL bottles can we get? $\frac{5000}{100}$ = 50 bottles of 100 mL each. Answer.

CHAPTER 11

DILUTION AND CONCENTRATION

11.1 Introduction.

Frequently pharmaceutical preparations are diluted or concentrated to achieve a given required concentration. We may have a 70 % alcohol solution, but for our purpose we may need to dilute it to 50%. We may have "stock solutions" made purposely with high concentration so as to be diluted when needed before use. Likewise, we may have a preparation that we want to make more concentrated than it is now. For example, Whitfield's ointment used on normal contains 3% salicylic acid. We may need to reduce the concentration to suit Albinos for example. Or we may need to make it more concentrated by adding the active ingredient salicylic acid so as to treat infections of palms or soles of feet which have a thicker and tougher skin.

Dilution is the addition or admixture with solutions of lower strength. On the other hand, **Concentration** is addition of active ingredients or by admixture with solutions or mixtures of greater strength or by evaporation.

There are two important rules:

1. When the *ratio strength* units are given, convert them to percentages.
2. Whenever *proportions parts* are given, before entering into calculations reduce to lowest term e.g. 60:40 and 3:2

11.2. RELATIONSHIP BETWEEN CONCENTRATION AND VOLUME

1. Dilute a solution to twice original volume, its concentration is halved. The active ingredient remains the same but is now contained in twice the volume.
2. Evaporate solution to half its original volume. The concentration shall double.

11.2.1 PRINCIPLES OF CALCULATIONS

The amount of active ingredient remaining constant, any change in the quantity of solution or mixture of solids is inversely proportional to concentration, provided that the total volume is summative. Sometimes admixing two liquids may result in contraction of the final volume e.g. when admixing alcohols.

As you may have noticed in the previous sections almost all problems can be solved by any of the proportion methods:

1. Inverse proportions: $\dfrac{Volume\ of\ liquid\ A}{Volume\ of\ liquid\ B} = \dfrac{Concnetration\ of\ liquid\ B}{concentration\ of\ Liquid\ A}$

$$\dfrac{V_a}{V_b} = \dfrac{C_b}{C_a}$$

2. (Quantity of liquid A) x (its Concentration) = (Quantity of liquid B) x (its concentration)

$$(Va)(Ca) = (Vb)(Cb)$$

This formula is very useful in determining the concentration or quantity of any given solution, when a known volume of a solution is diluted or concentrated.

Q185. 400 mL of a 20% w/v solution are diluted to 2 liters. What is the resulting % strength of the diluted solution?	$Va = 400\ mL$. $Vb = 2\ L = 2000\ mL$ $Ca = 20\%$ $Cb =$ Unknown percent (which is asked) Method 1: $\dfrac{Va}{Vb} = \dfrac{Cb}{Ca}$ $\dfrac{400\ mL}{2000\ mL} = \dfrac{Cb\%}{20\%}$ $Cb = 4\%$ Answer. Method 2: $(Va)(Ca) = (Vb)(Cb)$ $400\ mL \times 20\% = 2000mL \times (Cb)$ $Cb = 4\%$ Answer Method 3: Calculate how much of the solute is contained in the first solution. In this case, 400 mL of a 20% solution. 20% w/v means that there are 20 g in 100 mL of solution. In 400 mL of a 20% solution there will be 80 g of solute. $\dfrac{20}{X} = \dfrac{100}{400}$ $X = \dfrac{400 \times 20}{100} = 80\ g$ Upon dilution, 80 g shall be in 2000 mL. The concentration shall be $\dfrac{80g}{2000\ mL} \times 100 = 4\%\ w/v$ Answer.
Q186. 250 mL of a 1:800 v/v solution are diluted to 1000 mL. What is the new strength?	Although we can work out this problem using Ratio Strength expression, it is convenient to work with percentage strength. We therefore recommend to firstly convert ratio strength to percent strength: $1{:}800 = \dfrac{1}{800} \times 100 = 0.125\%$ Then proceed as instructed above Method 1. $\dfrac{Va}{Vb} = \dfrac{Cb}{Ca}$ $\dfrac{250\ mL}{1000\ mL} = \dfrac{x\ \%}{0.125\ \%}$ $X = 0.03125\%$ But the question asks the new ratio strength and not the percent strength. We have to convert percentage into ratio strength: $\dfrac{0.03125\ g}{100\ mL} = \dfrac{1}{X}$ $X = \dfrac{100 \times 1}{0.03125} = 3200$ Thus The new ratio strength is 1:3200 Answer

	Method 2. $\frac{Va}{Vb} = \frac{Cb}{Ca}$ $\frac{250\ mL}{1000\ mL} = \frac{\frac{1}{X}}{\frac{1}{800}} = \frac{\left(\frac{1}{800}\right)(250)}{1000} = 0.0003125$ $X = \frac{1}{0.0003125} = 3200$ The ratio strength = 1:3200. Answer. **Method 3.** $(Va)(Ca) = (Vb)(Cb)$ $250\ mL \times 0.125\% = 2000\ mL \times X\%$ $X = \frac{250 \times 0.125}{1000} = 0.03125\% = 1:3200\ w/v$
Q187. If a 0.067% (w/v) lotion is diluted with equal quantity of water, what will be the ratio strength of the resulting lotion?	If the lotion was diluted with an equal quantity of water, it means its volume was doubled. If the initial volume was V, then the final volume after dilution is 2V If $Va = V$, then $Vb = 2V$ $Ca = 0.067\%$ Cb is unknown **Method 1.** $(Va)(Ca) = (Vb)(Cb)$ $V \times 0.067 = 2V \times Cb$ $Cb = \frac{V \times 0.067}{2V}$ V cancels itself, then $Cb = \frac{0.067}{2} = 0.0335\%\ w/v$ $0.0335\% = 1:300\ w/v$ Answer. **Method 2.** We can also take the initial volume of the lotion to be 100 mL. After dilution with an equal amount of water, the new volume becomes 200 mL. In the initial lotion, the concentration is 0.067%, which means there is 0.067 g of active constituent in 100 mL of the lotion. This amount when contained in 200 mL. the new concentration is $\frac{0.067}{200} \times 100 = 0.0335\% = 1:300$
Q188. What is the strength of Sodium chloride solution obtained by evaporating 800g of a 10% (w/v) solution to 250g?	Initial quantity, $Va = 800\ g$ Final quantity $Vb = 250\ g$ Initial concentration, $Ca = 10\%\ w/v$ Calculate the final concentration, Cb Applying $(Va)(Ca) = (Vb)(Cb)$ $800 \times 10 = 250 \times Cb$ $Cb = \frac{800\ g \times 10\ \%}{250\ g} = 32\%$

Q.189. How many mL of 1:5000 w/v solution of a drug can be made from 125 mL of a 0.2 % solution?	**Method 1:** Convert 1:5000 into percent strength
	$1:5000 = 0.02\%$
	$Ca = 0.2\%$ $Va = 125\,mL$
	$Cb = 1:5000 = 0.02\%$ Vb is unknown
	
	Apply the equation $(Va)(Ca) = (Vb)(Cb)$
	    $125\,mL \times 0.2\% = Vb \times 0.02\%$
	                                 $Vb = \frac{125\,mL \times 0.2\%}{0.02\%} = 1250\,mL$ Answer
	
	Method 2. If you wish you can work with ratio strength. Convert the initial concentration 0.2% into ratio strength
	$0.2\% = \frac{0.2}{100} = \frac{1}{X}$ $X = 500$ therefore $0.2\% = 1:500$
	
	$$(Va)(Ca) = (Vb)(Cb)$$
	
	$$125 \times \frac{1}{500} = Vb \times \left(\frac{1}{5000}\right)$$
	
	$$Vb = \frac{125 \times \frac{1}{500}}{\frac{1}{5000}} = 1250\,mL$$
	
	Method 2: $\frac{Va}{Vb} = \frac{Cb}{Ca}\frac{125}{Vb} = \frac{\frac{1}{500}}{\frac{1}{5000}}Vb = 1250\,mL$
	
	Method 3: Find the amount of active ingredient contained in
	                125 mL of a 0.2% solution.
	                0.2% means that there are 0.2 g in 100 mL. Therefore
	                in 125 mL there will be $\frac{0.2}{100} \times 125 = 0.25g$
	
	         If the concentration of the final solution is 1:5000,
	         It means that there is 1 g in 5000 mL. we need to find out in
	         how many mL will 0.25 g be contained.
	
	        $\frac{1}{5000} = \frac{0.25}{X}$ $X = 5000 \times 0.25 = 1250\,mL$ Answer.

Q190. Belladona leaf has been assayed as containing 0.40% w/w/ alkaloids. We need 150 g of belladona leaves to prepare 1 liter of Belladona tincture. How many grams shall we need if we want to prepare 5 liters?	If 150 g are in 1 liter, how many g are in 5 liters? $\frac{150g}{1000\,mL} = \frac{Xg}{5000\,mL}$ $X = 750\,g$ Answer

Q191. If we have belladonna leaf whose assay shows 0.45% w/w alkaloids, how much of this leaf do we need to obtain the same concentration?	The concentration of alkaloids in the first leaf is 0.40%. If the present leaf is 0.45%, let us find out how much is equivalent: $(Va)(Ca) = (Vb)(Cb)$ $150 \times 0.40\% = Vb \times 0.45\%$ $Vb = 133.33$ g. Then using the same analogy, $\frac{133.3}{1000} = \frac{X}{5000}$ $X = 666.65$g Answ. OR if 133.33g has same effect as 150 g, how much has the same effect as 750 g? $\frac{133.33}{150} \times 750 = 666.65$ g Answer.

11.3 DILUTION AND CONCENTRATION OF SOLIDS AND SEMISOLIDS

The Same principles as applied in the dilution and concentration of liquids also apply to dilution and concentration of solids and semisolids.

Q191. How many grams of lactose and how many milligrams of atropine sulphate should be used to make 4 g of 10%w/w atropine sulphate?	10%w/w means 10 g in 100 g. let us calculate how many g are in 4 g: $\frac{10 g}{X g} = \frac{100 g}{4 g}$ $X = 0.4$ g $= 400$ mg If in 4 g there is 0.4 g atropine, how many g of lactose are required? $4 g - 0.4 g = 3.6 g$ Therefore, we need 400 mg of Atropine sulphate and 3.6 g of lactose to make 4 g of 10% atropine sulphate. Answer
Q 192. How many grams of white Petroleum Jelly should be added to 300 g of a 50% Ichthamol to make a 10 % ointment?	$(Va)(Ca) = (Vb)(Cb)$ Or $\frac{Va}{Vb} = \frac{Cb}{Ca}$ $Va = 300$ g $\quad Ca = 50\%$ $Vb =$ Unknown $\quad Cb = 10\%$ $300 \times 50 = Vb \times 10 \quad Vb = 1500$ g Therefore, in order to make a 10% ointment from 300 g of 50% ointment we need to add 1500 g $- 300$ g $= 1200$ g of white petroleum jelly. Answer.
Q193. A sample of Opium contains 10% morphine and 30% moisture. Calculate the quantity of morphine that can be extracted from 400 g of this sample.	400g x 10% = 400 g x $\frac{10}{100}$ = 40g of morphine Answer.

Q194. If the sample of opium in the previous question was dried, how many g would it weigh?	The sample contains 30% moisture. When dried it would weigh 70% of the original weight = $400 \times \frac{70}{100} = 280\ g$ Answer
Q195. A fresh crude drug contains 9.8% of active ingredient and 25% water. What would be the percentage of active ingredient when it is dried?	100 g of fresh drug contains 25 g of water and 9.8 g active ingredient. When it is dried therefore it would weigh 75 g, but the active ingredient will remain to be 9.8 g The percentage of active ingredient = $\frac{9.8}{75} \times 100$ = **13.07% Answer**
Q196. A sample of opium contains 30% moisture and 10% morphine. How many grams of morphine could be obtained from 500 grams of dry opium?	500 g of dry opium = 70% of raw opium. How much is 100%? Thus raw opium = $500 \times \frac{100}{70} = 714.3\ g$ If morphine is 10% in raw opium, then from 714.3 of raw opium we can obtain **71.43 grams** of morphine. **Method 2:** 500 g of dry opium is equivalent to $\frac{500}{X} = \frac{70}{100}$ X = 714.3 fresh (undried) opium 10% of 714.3 = $714.3 \times \frac{10}{100} = 71.43\ g$

Q197.
℞ Zinc Oxide 1.5 g
   Starch 3.0 g
   White soft Paraffin ad 40.0g
 	
What is the percentage of Zinc oxide in this preparation?
	There is 1.5 g of zinc oxide in 40 g of the preparation. The % = $\frac{1.5}{40} \times 100 = 3.75\%$ **Answer**

Q198. If in the previous question you are asked to make the concentration of Zinc Oxide to be 15%, how many grams of Zinc oxide would you need?	Find out how many grams of zinc oxide are required to make 15% in 40 g of ointment: $\frac{15\ g}{x\ g} = \frac{100\ g}{40\ g}$ X = 6 But we already have 1.5 g zinc oxide. We therefore still need 6-1.5 = 4.5 g ZnO Answer.

Q199.
 	
℞ Zinc Oxide, finely sifted 6.0 g
  Coal Tar 6.0 g
  Emulsifying wax 5.0 g
  Starch 38.0 g
	First of all, find how many grams of the ingredients in 1.5 kg of ointment.
	1.5 kg = 1500 g
	The conversion factor = $\frac{1500}{100} = 15$
	The formula then becomes:
	  Zinc oxide = 6x 15 =90 g

Yellow soft paraffin   45.0 g
 	
Coal tar in the above formula is 6%. How much coal tar should be added to 1.5 kg of this preparation to make it 25%w/w?
	Coal tar = 6 x 15 = 90 g
	Emulsifying wax = 5 x 15 = 75 g
	Starch = 38 x 15 = 570 g
	Yellow Soft Paraffin 45 x 15 = 675 g
	
	Thus already there are 90 g of coal tar. The rest of ingredients constitute (90 +75+570+675 g) = 1410 g
	This is the diluents of the preparation, equivalent to 75% (the active ingredient is 25%)
	
	$\frac{75}{25} = \frac{1410}{X}$ $X = 470$ g of coal tar in 25% ointment.
	
	But we already have 90 g. Therefore, we still need 470-90 = 380 g. Answer.
	
	The formula becomes:
	   Zinc oxide 90 g
	   Coal tar 470 g
	   Emulsifying wax 75 g
	   Starch570 g
	   Yellow Soft Paraffin 675 g
	
	Method 2: Use your knowledge of algebra;
	
	In 1500 g, Coal tar is 90g, and the rest of ingredients constitute 1410 g
	
	Let that amount of Coal tar to be added in order to achieve a 25% ointment be X
	
	Then in order to have a 25% product, total amount of coal tar = X + 90; and the total ingredients = 1410 + X + 90
	
	$$\frac{X + 90}{(1410 + X + 90)} = \frac{25}{100}$$
	
	$100(x + 90) = 25 (1410 + X + 90)$
	
	Solving for X = 380. Answer

Q200. How many grams of zinc oxide should be added to 3400 g of a 15 % zinc oxide ointment to prepare a product containing 20% of zinc oxide?	3400g of 15% zinc oxide contain: 15% Zinc oxide $=\frac{3400 \times 15}{100} = 510\ g$ 85% base $= 3400 \frac{x85}{100} = 2890\ g$ In the 20% preparation, the base shall be 80% Thus 2890 g − 80%. Calculate what is 20%:

	By proportion: $\frac{80}{20} = \frac{2890}{x}$ $X = 722.5 \, g$ Therefore, zinc oxide to be added = 722.5 − 510 = 212.5 g Answer. ** *This problem can also be solved by the method of alligation alternate. See Q236*
Q201. How many grams of zinc oxide should be added in 765 g starch to make 25% Zinc Oxide Paste	25% zinc oxide paste contains ZnO 25% and starch 75% This means that 756 g of starch = 75% of the preparation. Calculate what is 25%: $\frac{75}{25} = \frac{765}{X}$ $X = 255 \, g$ Answer

11.4 TRITURATION OF POWDERS

Compounding of pharmaceutical preparation need accuracy and precision. It is not advisable to weigh less than 100 mg of a medicine unless you are using a high grade analytical balance. For very potent medicines (medicines which are so strong that they are used in minute quantities) the minimum allowable measurement is 300 mg. Amounts smaller than the recommended weighable amounts are obtained by making triturations.

Trituration means "diluting potent medicinal substances with an inert substance" usually lactose. Usually triturations are prepared by diluting one part by weight of finely powdered medicinal substance with nine parts by weight of finely powdered lactose. Therefore, triturations are essentially 1:10 w/w (or10%) mixtures. In order to obtain 15 mg of codeine phosphate for example, weigh 100 mg codeine phosphate and add 900 mg lactose (to make 1000 mg trituration). Mix properly. This is a 1:10 dilution whereby 150 mg of the trituration contains 15 mg of codeine phosphate.

Q202. Prepare and send 5 caps each containing 0.6 mg hyoscine hydrobromide	We need to prepare 5 capsules of hyoscine in at least 100 mg diluents for accuracy of measurement. For this potent medicine, whose dose is 0.6 mg (less than 50mg), it is not advisable to weigh less than 300 mg on a dispensing balance. (Smaller weights can be weighed if an analytical balance is available). We need to prepare portions of 150 mg each to contain 0.6 mg of active ingredient. Therefore, we may prepare a total 750mg, which shall contain 3 mg of hyoscine. Still this measurement is not possible because we cannot weigh 3 mg. Even if this amount was to be multiplied by 10 so that we prepare 7500 mg, still we shall have to weigh 30mg, which cannot be done accurately! Therefore, we may prepare 75000 mg whereby Weigh 300 mg Hyoscine hydro bromide and

	Mix with <u>74700mg</u> Lactose
	75000 mg mixture
	Take 150mg, which contains 0.6 mg of hyoscine. THIS IS NOT REMLOMMENDABLE because it would be very difficult to distribute the small amount in medicament evenly throughout the bulk of diluents.
	
	The proper procedure would be:
	Mix 300mg hyoscine Habra
	With 4700 mg Lactose
	        5000 mg (containing 6 mg Hyoscine HBr in each 100 mg)
	Take 300 mg (which contain 18 mg Hycoscine HBr)
	
	Mix 300 mg of the triturate above
	With 4200 mg lactose
	        4500 mg (containing 0.4 mg Hyoscine HBr in each 100 mg)
	Pack 150 mg amounts (each pack shall have 0,6 mg Hyoscine HBr)

Q203. Prepare a 1:10 trituration of atropine sulphate. How much of this trituration shall contain 25 mg?	In order to prepare this trituration, mix 150 mg atropine sulphate with 1350 mg lactose to make 1500 mg trituration of 1:10 w/w 25 mg = 0.025 g 10 g of this triturate has 1 g atropine sulphate How much has 0.025 g? $\frac{10\,g}{X\,g} = \frac{1\,g}{0.025\,g}$ X= 0.25 g Answer
How many grams of the trituration contains 5000µg atropine sulphate?	5000µg = 5 mg = 0.005g $\frac{10\,g}{X\,g} = \frac{1\,g}{0.005\,g}$ X = 0.05g Answer.
Q204. How many grams of atropine sulphate triturate (10%w/w) should be used to prepare 1 liter of solution containing 30mg per teaspoonful?	1 teaspoonful = 5 mL = 1 dose In 500 mL there will be $\frac{500}{5}$ = 100 doses Each dose has 30 mg. The total dose = 30mg x 100 = 3000 mg = 3 g For the 10% trituration it means there is 1 g atropine per 10 g trituration. Calculate how much shall have 3000 mg (= 3g)? $\frac{1}{3} = \frac{10}{X}$ X = 30 g Answer.

Q205. Calculate the quantity in grams of a 10% trituration of colchicine needed to prepare 200 capsules each of which containing 500 µg colchicine	Total amount of colchicine required = 200 capsules x 500 µg
	                                                             = 100000µg = 100 mg
	                                                             = 0.1 g
	
	A 10% trituration contains 1 g colchicine in 10 g trituration
	Calculate the quantity containing 0.1g colchicine:
	
	$\frac{1}{0.1} = \frac{10}{X}$ X = 10x0.1=1 g Answer.

11.5 STOCK SOLUTIONS

Stock solutions are solutions or relatively high concentration, usually prepared in bulk, from which smaller volumes can be dispensed quickly when required, and should be diluted to a specified ratio to provide the medicine in the required therapeutic concentration.

When a preparation is required to be dispensed in a large quantity, it is inconvenient to store (it needs a large storage space) or to carry when dispensed to a patient. For example, potassium permanganate bath, used as an antiseptic is required in the concentration of 1:1000w/v. At this concentration one may require 5 Liters! Such a large volume would be inconvenient for a patient to carry. Therefore, such a solution is prepared as a stock solution, with a high concentration. The volume of the stock solution is relatively small, convenient to store or to carry. When needed, it will be diluted in a specific proportion to provide the required concentration for use.

Potent substances are required in very minute amount which are difficult to measure or to weigh. A properly prepared stock solution permits the pharmacist to obtain accurately a quantity of solid or liquid which might otherwise be difficult to measure or weigh accurately.

Frequently prescribed salts solutions are also frequently prepared as stock solutions to provide the required amount without the necessity of weighing and dissolving it all the time.

Stock solutions are prepared on the basis of w/v and their concentrations are expressed as Ratio Strength or Percent (%)Strength. They must be properly labeled to display their concentration, e.g. .... mL = 1 mL or %, by parts, ratio strength, 100mL = 1g etc.

You may be asked to calculate the amount of solution of a given strength to be used to prepare a solution of desired amount and strength, or to actually prepare it. You must therefore be prepared to perform such tasks.

Q206. Burrow's solution has 5% Aluminium acetate. How many liters of Burrow's solution should be used to prepare 1 liter of a 1:800 w/v solution for use as wet dressing?	*For convenience sake, change ratio strength to percentage strength:* $1:800 = 1/800 \times 100 = 0.125\%$ $Ca = 5\%$, Va is unknown $Cb = 0.125\%$, $Vb = 1\,L = 1000\,mL$ **Method 1:** $(Va)(Ca) = (Vb)(Cb)$ $\quad Va\,(L) \times 5\% = 1000\,(mL) \times 0.125\%$ $\quad Va = \dfrac{1000 \times 0.125}{5} \qquad Va = 25\,mL$ **Method 2:** $\dfrac{Va}{Vb} = \dfrac{Cb}{Ca}\;\dfrac{Va\,(L)}{1\,(L)} = \dfrac{0.125\%}{5\%} \quad Va = 0.025L = 25mL$ **Method 3:** Calculate quantity of active ingredient in the final solution and then find out how much of the original solution will have that quantity: 1: 800 means that there is 1 g of active constituent in 800 mL of solution. How many g shall be in the required amount of 1 liter: $\dfrac{1g}{X\,g} = \dfrac{800\,mL}{1000\,mL} \quad X = 1.25g.$ The original solution is 5%, which means there are 5 g in 100 mL of solution. How much shall hold 1.25 g?

	$\frac{5\,g}{1.25\,g} = \frac{100\,mL}{X\,mL}$	$X = \frac{1.25 \times 100}{5} = 25\,mL$
Q207. How many mL of 1:400 w/v stock solution is needed to make 4 liters of 1:2000 w/v solution?	$1:400 = 0.25\%,\ 1:2000 = 0.05\%$ $Ca = 0.25\%;\quad Cb = 0.05\%$ Va is the unknown parameter; $Vb = 4\,L = 4000\,mL$ **Method 1:** $(Va)(Ca) = (Vb)(Cb)$ $4000 \times 0.05 = Vb \times 0.25\quad Vb = \frac{4000 \times 0.05}{0.25} = 800\,mL$ Answer. **Method 2:** $\frac{Va}{Vb} = \frac{Cb}{Ca} \quad \frac{4\,(L)}{Vb\,(L)} = \frac{0.25\,\%}{0.05\,\%} \quad Vb = \frac{0.05 \times 4}{0.25} = 0.8\,L$ $\hspace{10cm}= 800\,mL$ **Method 3:** Calculate amount of ingredient contained in 4000 mL of a 1:2000 w/v solution: $\frac{1\,g}{X} = \frac{2000\,mL}{4000\,mL}\quad X = 2\,g$. If the original solution is 1:400 by concentration, it means there is 1 g of active ingredient in 400 mL solution. We need therefore to calculate how many mL will contain the 2 g: $\frac{1\,g}{2\,g} = \frac{(400\,mL)}{V}\quad V = 800\,mL$	
Q208. We have in stock a 1% official red coloring agent. How much of this agent should be used in preparation of 450 mL of Amphogel, given the following formula? Certified red dye 1:10000 Amphogel ad 180 mL	**Method 1:** The concentration of the red dye in the final preparation is 1:10000, this means that there is 1 g in 10000 mL of the solution. We are asked to prepare 450 mL. Let us calculate how much of the dye is needed in this quantity: $\frac{1\,g}{Xg} = \frac{10000\,mL}{450\,mL}\quad X = 0.045\,g$ The dye is available as 1%, which means 1 g in 100 mL of solution. Let us find out how many mL shall contain the required 0.45g of the dye: $\frac{1}{0.045} = \frac{100}{x}\quad X = 4.5\,mL$ **Method 2:** $(Va)(Ca) = (Vb)(Cb)$ $\hspace{2cm}Ca = 1\%,\ Va = Unknown,\ Vb = 450\,mL,$ $\hspace{2cm}Cb = 1:10,000 = 0.01\%$ $Vu\,(mL) \times 1\% = 450\,(mL) \times 0.01\%\quad Va = \frac{450 \times 0.01}{1} = 4.5\,mL.$	

Q209	Change 1:50 in two percent strength. $1/50 \times 100 = 2\%$

℞:   Ephedrine sulphate   0.25%
        Rose water ad   60 mL
        Sig: for Nose
 	
 How many mL of stock solution of 1:50 ephedrine sulphate is needed?
	Method 1: Calculate how much ephedrine sulphate is contained in the 60 mL of the preparation:
	 $60 \, g \times \frac{0.25}{100} = 0.15 \, g$ of ephedrine sulphate needed.
	 If the stock solution is 1:50, it means there is 1 g of ephedrine sulphate in 50 mL of solution. We need to find out how many ML shall provide 0.15 g
	 $\frac{1\,g}{0.15\,g} = \frac{50\,mL}{X\,mL}$ $X = 7.5 \, mL$ Answer.
	
	 Method 2: $\frac{Va}{Vb} = \frac{Cb\ 60\,mL}{Ca\ x\,mL} = \frac{(2\,\%)}{0.25\,\%}$ $X = 7.5 \, mL$ Answer.

CALCULATIONS REQUIRED TO PREPARE STOCK SOLUTIONS: FIND THE QUANTITY OF ACTIVE INGREDIENT IN A SPECIFIC AMOUNT OF SOLUTION TO MAKE A DILUTED SOLUTION

Sometimes you are required to prepare a strong solution to dispense to a patient so that the patient is instructed to dilute it to appropriate therapeutic concentration in a specified ratio. The calculations involved are described below.

| Q210. How much silver nitrate is needed to prepare 200 mL of stock solution, so that 5 mL diluted to 500 mL yields 1:1000 solution? | *This kind of a problem is worked "backward"! We start from the final solution to work out what the initial Stock solution should be.*
 The strength of dilute solution gives the quantity of active ingredient that the strong solution must have contained. Then by proportion calculate how much active ingredient must be present in any amount of stock solution.

 Step 1: Determine how many grams are in 500 mL of a 1:1000 solution.
 1:1000 means that 1000mL contain 1 g silver nitrate.
 500 mL will have 0.5 g

 [This may also be expressed as $1:1000::X:500$, $X = 0.5$]

 Step 2: Determine how much should be in the stock solution.

      This same 0.5 g is the quantity of silver nitrate in 5 mL of the stronger solution, or the stock solution that we are supposed to prepare. If 0.5 g are in 5 mL, how much is in 200 mL?

 $\frac{5\,mL}{200\,mL} = \frac{0.5\,g}{X\,g}$ $X = \frac{200 \times 0.5}{5} = 20g$ Answer.

 [dissolve 20 g silver nitrate in enough water to make a 200 mL solution] |

Q211. How much of a drug is needed to make 240 mL of a solution such that when a teaspoon is diluted to 1 liter, a 1:2000 solution results?	**The question requires you to prepare a solution that will be dispensed to a patient with instructions that "Add one teaspoonful (5 mL) of this solution to water so as to make 1 liter of solution". 1 liter = 1000 mL **Step 1** Determine how many g are in 1 liter of a 1:2000 solution. $\frac{1\,(g)}{X\,(g)} = \frac{2000\,mL}{1000\,mL}$ $X = ½\,g = 0.5\,g$ **Step 2** The 0.5 g in the dilute solution came from the 5 mL (teaspoonful) of the original stock solution (prescription order). WE can use the following proportion: $\frac{0.5\,g}{X\,g} = \frac{5\,mL}{240\,mL}$ $X = 24g.$ Add 24 g to enough water to make a 240 mL solution. Answer.
Q212. How many mL of water should be added to 375 mL of 1:250 solution of Cetrimide to make a 1:5000 solution?	**Method 1:** **Step 1:** Convert ratio strength to percent strength to simplify calculation (if you are comfortable you may make work with ratio strength) $1:250 = \frac{1}{250} \times 100 = 0.4\%$ $1:5000 = \frac{1}{5000} \times 100 = 0.02\%$ **Step 2** This is a normal dilution, whereby 375 mL of 0.4 % solution are diluted to make a 0.02% solution. Calculate the volume of the new dilute solution, then find the difference between dilute and strong solution. $Va \times Ca = Vb \times Cb$ $Ca = 0.4\%, Va = 375\,mL$ $Cb = 0.02\%\ Vb = unknown$ (or required) $375 \times 0.4 = Vb \times 0.02$ $Vb = 7500\,mL$ **Step 3:** In order to find how much water should be added, find the difference between the volume of diluted solution prepared and the volume of stronger (stock) solution. $Vb - Va = 7500 - 375mL = 7125mL$ Add 7125 mL of water to 375 mL of the stronger solution to obtain 7500 mL of the weaker solution. Answer. **Method 2:** Calculate the quantity of ingredient in the strong solution (375 mL of 1:250) $\frac{1}{250} \times 375 = 1.5\,g$ The dilute solution is 1:5000, which means 1 g is in 5000 mL. Find the amount that can accommodate 1.5 g: $\frac{1}{1.5} = \frac{5000}{X}$ $X = 7500.$ Water to be added = 7500-375 = 7125mL Answer.

Q213 ℞: Benzalkonium Cl solution 240 mL Make a solution such that 10 mL diluted to one liter equals 1:5000 solution Sig: 10 mL diluted to one liter. For Ext. Use only. How many mL of 17% solution of benzalkonium Chloride solution should be used in compounding this prescription?	The final solution (diluted solution) is 1 liter (1000mL) of 1:5000. 1:5000 means 1 g in 5000 mL solution. Find how many g are in 1000 mL: $\frac{5000 \, mL}{1000 \, mL} = \frac{1 \, g}{X \, g}$ $X = 0.2$ g benzalkonium chloride in 1 L This is the same amount in 10 mL of the "stronger" solution. If 0.2 g of Benzalkonium Cl is in 10 mL; how many g are in 240 mL? $\frac{10 \, mL}{240 \, mL} = \frac{0.2g}{Xg}$ $X = 4.8$ mL Since 17 % concentrate contains 17 g in 100 mL, how many mL shall have 4.8g? $\frac{17g}{4.8g} = \frac{100mL}{XmL}$ $X = 28.2$ mL Answer.
Q214. What weight of potassium permanganate is required to produce 500 mL of solution such that 25 mL of this solution diluted to half liter gives 0.025% w/v solution?	The final solution is 0.025% which means 100 mLs of the solution contains 0.025 g potassium permanganate. Thus in 500 mLs there are 0.025 x 5 = 0.125g potassium permanganate. This is the same amount which was in 25 mLs used to dilute the solution. Thus in 500 mLs of the original solution there should be $\frac{0.125 \times 500}{25} = 2.5$ g and this is the amount of potassium permanganate required to make the original 500 mL solution. Ans.
Q215. How many milliliters of water should be added to 100mL of a 1:100 (w/v) Dettol solution such that 25 mL diluted with 25 mL of water will yield a 1:400 (w/v) Dettol solution?	The final solution is 1:400 = $\frac{1}{400}$ x 100= 0.25% In 25 mL of the final solution there are $\frac{0.25}{100}$ x 25 = 0.0625g This is the amount which was in 25 mL of the diluting Dettol solution. To find the strength we need to calculate the quantity in 100 mL. Thus if 0.0625 g is in 25 mL, how many grams are in 100 mL? $\frac{0.0625}{X} = \frac{25}{100}$ $X = 0.25$g Dettol. Or 0.25% 1:100 solution is 1% ($\frac{1}{100}$ x1 = 1%) Therefore, in order for it to be 0.25% more water should be added. (Va)(Ca) = (Vb)(Cb) Va = 100 mL, Ca = 1% Vb = unknown Cb = 0.25% 1% x 100 = 0.25% x Vb Vb = 400 mL Thus add 300 mL to 100 mL of 1:100 solution to make 400mL of 0.25% solution.

11.6 DILUTION OF ALCOHOLS

When water is added to or mixed with alcohol, the total volume diminishes, because there is contraction. Therefore, we cannot use the % v/v strength. However, the volume contraction does not affect weight. Thus we can find the weight of water (and therefore volume) needed to dilute alcohol to a desired w/w.

Q216. How much water should be added to 2.5L of 85% v/v alcohol to prepare 50% v/v alcohol?	$(Va)(Ca) = (Vb)(Cb)$ $Va = 2.5\ L = 2500\ mL;\ \ Ca = 85\%$ $Vb = Unknown\ \ \ \ \ \ Cb = 50\%$ $2500\ mL \times 85\% = Vb\ mL \times 50\%$ $Vb = \frac{2500 \times 85}{50}$ $\ \ \ \ \ \ \ \ \ Vb = 4250\ mL$ Therefore, Add enough water to 2.5L of 85% alcohol to make 4250 mL. Answer.

Q217.
℞: Chloroform Liniment   60 mL
    Methylsalicylate   60 mL
    Alcohol 80%   ad   240 mL
Sig: Apply to affected area
 	
80% alcohol is not available, but we have 95% alcohol in the store. How many mL of 95%v/v alcohol and how much water should be used to prepare the prescription?
	Already Chloroform Liniment and Methylsalicylate contribute 60 mL + 60 mL = 120 mL. For the total volume of the prescription to be made we need to make it to 120 mL.
	
	Another way of asking this question is: How many mL of 95% alcohol are required to make 120 mL of 80% alcohol?
	
	$(Va)(Ca) = (Vb)(Cb)$
	$120 \times 80 = Vb \times 95$ $\ \ \ \ Vb = \frac{120 \times 80}{95} = 101.05\ mL\ approx\ 101.1$
	
	Therefore, add enough water to 101.1 mL of 95% alcohol to make 120 mL, then add the rest of ingredients. Answer.

Q218. Prepare 70% alcohol for use as a disinfectant given 350mL of 95% alcohol	This question is the same as how many mL of water should be added to 350mL of 95% alcohol to make 70% alcohol: $(Va)(Ca) = (Vb)(Cb)$ $\ \ \ \ \ \ \ \ \ \ Ca = 95\%,\ \ Va = 350\ mL,$ $\ Cb = 70\%.\ \ \ Vb= Unknown$ $95 \times 350 = 70 \times Vb$ $\ \ \ \ \ Vb = 475\ mL$ Add enough water to 350 mL of 95% alcohol to make 475 mL of 70% alcohol. Answer.

11.7 MIXING MIXTURES SOLIDS OR LIQUIDS OF DIFFERENT STRENGTHS

11.7.1 ALLIGATION MEDIAL AND ALLIGATION ALTERNATE

You may wish to mix solutions or ointments of different strengths to obtain a certain concentration. This concentration shall be somewhere between the strength of the solution with higher strength and that of the solution of lower strength. A method of solving problems that involve the mixing of solutions or mixtures of solids possessing different percentage strengths is called **Alligation**. There are two such methods, namely **Alligation medial** and **Alligation alternate**.

Alligation medial is a method that is used to calculate the concentration of a liquid obtained by mixing solutions or solid mixtures of different percent strengths. The resultant percent strength is actually a "weighted average" of other constituent's strengths.

Alligation Medial finds use when you are asked to **calculate the percent strength of a mixture that has been made by mixing two or more components of given percent strengths.** Let us follow the example below:

Q219. Mix 400 mL of 30% alcohol, 5000 mL of 45% alcohol and 1200 mL of 70% alcohol. What is the new concentration of alcohol?	*Step 1: Determine the total amount of the active ingredient in the mixture:* 400 mL of 30% alcohol contain $400 \times \frac{30}{100} = 120\ mL$ alcohol. 5000 mL of 45 % alcohol contain $5000 \times \frac{45}{100} = 2250\ mL$ alcohol 1200 mL of 70% alcohol contain $1200 \times \frac{70}{100} = 840\ mL$ alcohol **Step 2.** Obtain total volume of mixture: $\quad$ 400 mL + 5000 mL + 1200 mL = $\quad$ 6600 mL **Step 3.** Determine the percent of alcohol in the mixture: $\quad$ Total alcohol = 120 mL + 2250 mL 840 mL = 3210 mL $\quad$ Total Volume = 6600 $\quad$ % alcohol = $\frac{3210}{6600} \times 100 = 48.6\%$ Answer.
Q220. What is the percentage of alcohol in a mixture made by mixing 3 liters of 30%, ½ L of 50% and 750 mL of 95% alcohol?	30% x 3000 mL = $\quad$ 900 mL 50 % x 500 mL = $\quad$ 250 mL 95% x $\underline{750\ mL}$ = $\underline{712.5mL}$ $\quad$ 4250 mL $\quad\quad$ 1862.5 mL New concentration = $\frac{1862.5}{4250} \times 100$ = 43.82% Alcohol. Answer. **Method 2 (shortcut):** You may obtain the new concentration by dividing the sum of (% strength x quantity) by the sum of (quantities): $\quad$ % $\quad\quad$ Quantities $\quad\quad$ % x Quantity $\quad$ 30 $\quad$ x $\quad\quad$ 3000 = $\quad\quad$ 90000 $\quad$ 50 $\quad$ x $\quad\quad$ 500 = $\quad\quad$ 25000 $\quad$ 95 $\quad$ x $\quad\quad$ $\underline{750}$ = $\quad\quad$ $\underline{71250}$ $\quad\quad\quad\quad\quad\quad$ 4250 $\quad\quad\quad\quad$ 186250 $\quad\quad$ The new concentration = $\quad\frac{\Sigma\ (C\ x\ Q)}{\Sigma\ (Q)}$ $\frac{186250}{4250}$ =43.82% Answer. ** *Using this method you do not multiply by 100 to obtain the percentage.*
The Concentration of the resultant solution or mixture is obtained by dividing the sum of the products obtained by multiplying a series of quantities by their respective concentrations by the total quantities summed together:	

$$\text{New concentration} = \frac{(C_1 \times Q_1) + (C_2 \times Q_2) + (C_3 \times Q_3) + \cdots (C_n \times Q_n)}{Q_1 + Q_2 + Q_3 + \cdots Q_n}$$

Where C_1, C_2, C_3, C_n = concentrations of individual solutions or mixtures;
$Q_1, Q_2, Q_3 \ldots Q_n$ = Quantities of Solution 1.2.3 up to n

OR $\quad$ New Concentration = $\dfrac{\text{Sum of product of concentration and quantity}}{\text{sum of Quantity}}$

$$= \frac{\Sigma\,(C \times Q)}{\Sigma\,(Q)}$$

Q221. What is the percentage of the following mixture? 1.5 L 30% alcohol, 3000 mL od 60% alcohol, 450 mL of 90% alcohol and 1 liter of water.	$1\,L = 1000\,mL$ $30 \times 1500 = 45000$ $60 \times 3000 = 18000$ $90 \times 450 = 40500$ $0 \times 1000 = 0$ (the concentration of alcohol in water is 0) $\overline{5950103500}$ Concentration of alcohol = $\dfrac{103500}{5950}$ = 17.4% Answer.
Q222. A pharmaceutical technician mixes 300 g of 15 % Ichthamol ointment, 500 g of 5% Icthamol ointment, 200 g of 20% Ichthamol ointment and 1 kg of white soft paraffin. Calculate the percent strength of the resulting product	$\begin{array}{cccl} C & Q & & C \times Q \\ 15 & \times\ 300 & = & 4500 \\ 5 & \times\ 500 & = & 2500 \\ 20 & \times\ 200 & = & 4000 \\ 0 & \times\ 1000 & = & 0 \text{ (concentration of ichthamol in}\\ & \ \ \ 2000 & & 11000 \ \ \text{yellow soft paraffin = 0\%)} \end{array}$ The new % strength = $\dfrac{\Sigma\,(C \times Q)}{\Sigma\,(Q)} = \dfrac{11000}{2000} = 5.5\%\,w/w$ Answer.
Q223. ℞: Phenobarbital Elixir 15 mL Aromatic Elixir 60 mL Belladona Tincture 25 mL Purified water Ad 125 mL Sig: tsp tid 7/7 Phenobarbital and Aromatic elixirs contain 15% and 22% alcohol respectively. Belladona tincture is 65% alcohol. Calculate the percentage of alcohol in the product.	Volume of water = (total volume − volume of the rest of ingredients) $= 125 - (15+60+25) = 125 - 100 = 25\,mL$ $\begin{array}{cccl} C\,\% & Q\,mL & & C \times Q \\ 15 & \times\ 15 & = & 225 \\ 22 & \times\ 60 & = & 1320 \\ 65 & \times\ 25 & = & 1625 \\ 0 & \times\ \underline{25} & = & \underline{0} \\ & \ \ \ 125 & & 3170 \end{array}$ Concentration of the product = $\dfrac{\Sigma\,(C \times Q)}{\Sigma\,(Q)}$ $= \dfrac{3170}{125} = 25.36\%\ v/v$ Answer
Q224. Three equal amounts of Benzoic acid ointment, containing 3%, 6% and 9% benzoic acid were mixed. Calculate the percent strength of the resulting	Let the volume of each ointment be V. Then $\begin{array}{l} 3 \times V = 3V \\ 6 \times V = 6V \\ 9 \times \underline{V} = \underline{9V} \\ 3V\ \ \ \ 18V \end{array}$ $\qquad \begin{array}{l} V+V+V = 3V \\ 3V + 6V + 9V = V(3+6+9) = 18V \end{array}$

mixture.	% strength = $\frac{18V}{3V}$ = 6% w/w Answer. ** You may also assume the amount of each ointment to be 100 g and work out the final concentration using this quantity for each of the ointments.

Q225.
℞
Coal tar solution
  (85% alcohol)... 64 mL
Glycerin ....128 mL
Alcohol (95%) ....400 mL
Boric acid solution
    Ad ....800 mL
 	
Sig: Apply bd 1/30
 	
What is the percentage of alcohol in this medication lotion?
	Volume of boric acid solution = 800 – (64 + 128 + 400)
	                            = 800 – 592 = 208 mL
	
	<u>Vol. (mL) % Volume x %</u>
	64 x 85 = 5440
	128 x 0 = 0
	400 x 95 = 38000
	<u>208</u> x 0 = <u> 0</u>
	800 43440
	
	% of alcohol = $\Sigma (C \times Q)$ = $\frac{43440}{800}$ = 54.3% Answer
	                  $\Sigma (Q)$

You may be asked to find out **proportions by which two or more solutions of mixtures having different strengths or concentration should be mixed to obtain a specific required strength.** In order to do this, you apply a method known as **Alligation alternate.** When we obtain these proportion or parts we can calculate the actual quantity that we may mix to obtain any desired concentration. The following rules are observed in this calculation:

1. When solutions or mixtures of different strengths are mixed, the resulting mixture has concentration **between** that of a **lower** concentration and that of a **higher** concentration. The mixture is stronger than the weaker solution but is weaker than the stronger solution. Thus the resulting strength is a "weighted average" of the constituting strengths.

2. The substance with a higher strength than that required is the one with a lower quantity.

3. The gain in value or amount of one substance balances the loss in value or amount of the other substance.

Q226. In what proportions should alcohol 10% be mixed with alcohol 80% to produce alcohol 50 %?	The 10% alcohol is 40% too weak compared to the required 50% (50-10), and the 80% is 30% too strong (80-50). The **difference between the strength of stronger solution and desired strength indicates the number of parts of the weaker strength** to be used, 80 – 50 = 30 parts of weaker solution while the **difference between the desired strength and the strength of the weaker solution indicates the number of parts of the**

stronger solution to be used 50 – 10 = 40 parts of the stronger solution.

This relationship is represented schematically as follows:

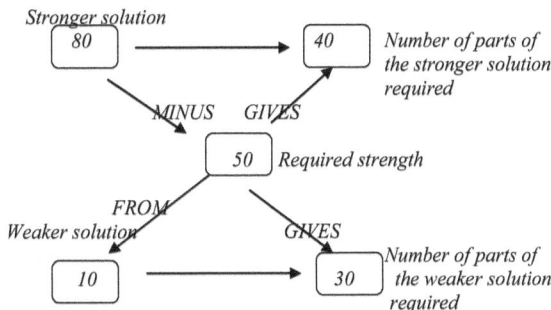

We need to mix 40 parts of 80% alcohol and 30 parts of 10% alcohol to make 50% alcohol. The proportions are 40:30 or simply 4:3

Strengths of **available** solutions are on **the left hand** side with the higher strength on top, while the lower strength is at the bottom. The **required strength** is placed in **the center**.
Subtract the required strength from the stronger concentration, and put the result on the right side opposite to the weaker strength. **These are number of parts of weaker** solution required. Then subtract the weaker strength from the required strength and place the results on the right side opposite the stronger solution. **These are number of parts of stronger** solution required

H%		x parts required
	R	
L%		y required

$x = R - L$
$y = H - R$

This can be proved mathematically as follows:

$Hx + Ly = R(x + y)$
$ = Rx + Ry$
Arrange similar values on one side: $Hx - Rx = Ry - Ly$

	$x(H-R) = y(R-L)$ $$\frac{y}{x} = \frac{H-R}{R-Y}$$ The name **Alligation** is derived from Latin *alligation* which means the act of attaching and hence refers to lines drawn during calculation to bind quantities together
Q227. In what proportions should 35% and 75% alcohol be mixed to make 500 mL of 65% alcohol? How many mL of 75% and how many mL of 35% alcohol should be mixed to make 500 mL of 65% alcohol?	75 ↘ ↗ 30 75 | 30 65 OR 65 35 ↗ ↘ 10 35 | 10 We need 30 parts of 75% alcohol and 10 parts of 35% alcohol or simply 3:1 proportions. Answer Total number of parts = 30 + 10 = 40 500 mL = 40 parts Amount of 75% alcohol required = $\frac{30}{40} \times 500 = 375\ mL$ Amount of 35% alcohol required = $\frac{10}{40} \times 500 = 125\ mL$
Q228. In what proportions should 20% zinc oxide ointment and white soft paraffin be mixed to prepare 15% zinc oxide ointment?	20 ↘ ↗ 15 15 0 ↗ ↘ 5 *(white soft paraffin has 0% zinc oxide)* The ratio of 20% ZnO ointment and Soft paraffin should be 15:5 or 3:1
Q229. How much white soft paraffin (a diluent) should be added to 20% Zinc oxide ointment to prepare 200 g of 15% Zinc oxide ointment?	$VaCa = VbCb$ $Va \times 20\% = 200 \times 15\%$ $Va = \frac{15 \times 200}{20} = 150$ This means that we need 150 g of 20% Zinc ointment and in order to get 200 g we add 50 g white soft paraffin. The ratio of 20% zinc oxide ointment to white soft paraffin is 150:50 = 3:1
You may mix more than two solutions or mixtures and calculate in what proportion the components	

should be mixed to obtain a desired concentration. The lots or preparations having stronger concentration than the required one are grouped together and linked to the required concentration. Likewise, the lots having weaker solution than the desired one are grouped together and linked to the required concentration.

Q230. In what proportions should 2% iodine, 3% iodine and 6% iodine be mixed to get 4.5% iodine	The 6% and 3% are linked together, because the required strength of 4.5% can be obtained by mixing such concentrations whereby the required strength is intermediate. Similarly, concentration 6% and 2 % can be linked. However, concentration 3% and 2% cannot be linked because the required concentration 4.5% cannot be obtained by mixing 3% and 2%!
	
	 Therefore, find out proportions in which 6% and 3% may be mixed:
	
	 6 1.5
	      4.5
	 3 1.5
	
	 Then find out proportions in which 6% and 2% may be mixed
	
	 6 2.5
	      4.5
	 2 1.5
	
	 Instead of working separately, link the possible combination and work together:
	
	 6 1.5 + 2.5 = 4 parts of 6% iodine
	 3 4.5 1.5 parts of 3% iodine
	 2 1.5 parts of 2% iodine
	
	 The proportion of 6%, 3% and 2% are 4:1.5:1.5 = 8:3:3
	
	 Check using allegation medial.
	 8 x 6 = 48
	 3 x 3 = 9
	 <u>3 x 2 =</u> <u>6</u>
	 14 63
	
	 $\frac{63}{14} = 4.5\%$

Q231. A supervisor asks a Pharmaceutical assistant to mix four lots of ichthamol paste containing 5%, 25%, 30 % and 50% ichthamol respectively so as to make 5 kg of 20% ichthamol ointment. Show how this task can be worked out.	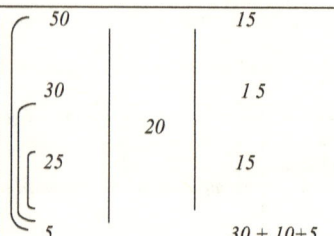
	The proportions are 15:15:15:45 = 3:3:3:9
	Check: 3 x 50 = 150
	         3 x 30 = 90
	         3 x 25 = 75
	<u>9 x 5 = 45</u>
	         18 360 $\frac{360}{18}$ = 20%
	5 kg of 20% Ichthamol are required. The proportions have been worked out as 3:3:3:9 for 50,30 25 and 5% ointment.
	Total parts = 3+3+3+9 = 18
	The respective quantities of ichthamol ointments required =
	$\frac{3}{18}$ x5000= 833.33
	$\frac{9}{18}$ x 5000 = 2500
	Thus Mix 833.33g of Ichthamol 50%, 833.33g Ichthamol 30%, 833.33 g Ichthamol 25% and 2500g of Ichthamol 5% to get 5000 g of Ichthamol 20% Answer.

Q232. In what proportions can we mix 20%, 15% 5% and 2% Sulphur ointment to produce 10% Sulphur ointment?	Each of a weaker ointment is linked or paired with a stronger one to obtain the desired strength. There are several ways in which this can be done. One of them is as follows: 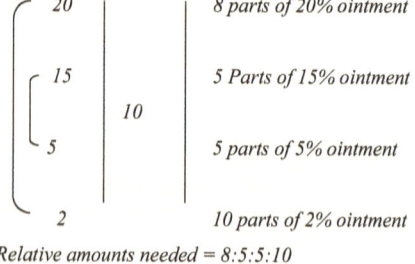 Relative amounts needed = 8:5:5:10

	Another way of pairing the ointments is:
	``
   ┌─ 20 ─────────────── 5 parts of 20% ointment
   │
   │ 15 ─────────────── 8 Parts of 15% ointment
   │   10
   └─ 5 ─────────────── 10 parts of 5% ointment

      2 ─────────────── 5 parts of 2% ointment
```
Relative amounts needed = 5:8:10:5 |
| Q233. You have been supplied with 800 g of 5% coal tar ointment, 1 kg of 10 % coal tar ointment and 500 mg of 10% zinc oxide paste. If these are mixed, calculate additional pure coal tar required to make the final ointment contain 15% coal tar. | Using alligation medial, calculate the total % of coal tar in the mixture:<br><br>800   x   5%   =    4000<br>1000  x   10%  =    10,000<br>_0.5_  x   0    =    ___0___ (zinc oxide paste has 0% coal tar)<br>1800.5              14.000<br><br>% coal tar in the mixture    =    _14,000_ = 7.78%<br>                                      1800.5<br>Using alligation alternate we can calculate how much coal tar is needed to make the final mixture 15%. Pure coal tar is 100%<br><br>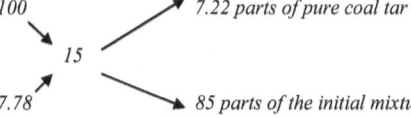<br><br>Total quantity of coal tar available after mixing the ointment = 1800.5 g, which is equivalent to 85 parts.<br>So how much is equivalent to how 7.22 parts?<br><br>$\frac{7.22 \text{ parts}}{85 \text{ parts}} = \frac{X}{1800.5}$   $X = \frac{1800.5 \times 7.22}{85} = 152.5$ g pure coal tar. Ans.<br><br>See also Q 199 above. |
| Q234. Melleril suspension is available as thioridazine 100 mg/mL and 25 mg/mL solutions. | 100 mg/mL = 100 x 100mg per 100 mL = 10g / 100 mL = 10%<br>25 mg /mL = 25 x 100 mg per 100mL = 2.5 g/100mL = 2.5%<br>75mg / mL = 75 x 100 mg per 100 mL  = 7.5 g /100mL =7.5% |
```

In what proportions should the two solutions be mixed to produce a solution containing 75 mg/mL thioridazine?	Using allegation alternate, 2.5 2.5 7.5 10 5.0 the ratio is 2.5: 5.0 = __1:2__

Q235. A pharmaceutical technician mixed 250 milliliters of each of 10% and 40% alcohols. But he needed a 50% alcohol. How many milliliters of such a solution (50% alcohol) could he make if he had enough 70% alcohol in his store?	Using alligation medial,
	250 mL x 10% = 2500
	250 mL x 40 % = 10000
	500 12500
	
	The resultant solution = $\frac{12500}{500}$ = 25%
	
	In order to find how much 70 % alcohol is needed to make 50% alcohol, use alligation alternate:
	70 25 parts of 70% alcohol
	      50
	25 20 parts of the initial solution
	
	20 parts are equivalent to 500mL (i.e. 250mL + 250 mL)
	
	Thus 25 parts are equivalent to $\frac{25 \times 500}{20}$ = 625 mL. of 70%. Ans
	
	Method 2: use alligation medial and algebraic knowledge:
	
	Let the volume of 70% alcohol be V
	
	Then 250 x 10 = 2500
	           250 x 40 = 10000
	           V x 70 = 70V
	
	% alcohol of the product = $\frac{2500 + 10{,}000 + 70V}{250+250+V}$ = 50%
	
	2500+10,000 +70V = 50(250+250+V)
	12500 +70 V = 50(500 +V) = 25000 + 50V
	70V-50V = 25,000 – 12,500
	20V = 12,500
	V = 625 mL Answer.

Q236. How many grams of zinc oxide should be added to 3400 g of a 15 % zinc oxide ointment to	Pure Zinc oxide is 100% in concentration. 100 5

prepare a product containing 20% of zinc oxide?	20 15　　　　　　80 Relative amounts of zinc oxide and zinc oxide ointment = 5:80 　　　　　　　　　　　　　　　　　　　　　　　　= 1:16 Thus 3400g = 16 parts. Let us calculate what is 1 part: $\frac{16}{1} = \frac{3400}{X}$　　　　　$X = 212.5$ g Answer **This problem could be solved by other methods. See Question Q200.**

11.7.2 ALLIGATION MEDIAL AND ALLIGATION ALTERNATE IN SPECIFIC GRAVITIES OF LIQUID MIXTURES

Alligation medial and Alligation alternate methods can be applied to solve problems involving specific gravities. When liquids of different specific gravities are nixed it is possible to calculate the specific gravity of the mixture provided there is no change in volume during or after mixing the liquids. Likewise, just like in solving problems involving concentrations, it is possible to determine the proportions in which two or more liquids of different specific gravities can be mixed to obtain any desired specific gravity.

Q237. What is the specific gravity of a mixture containing ½ liter glycerin (Specific Gravity = 1.250), 2.5 L of alcohol (specific gravity = 0.810 and 1.5 L water (specific gravity = 1.000)? Assume no change in volume.	To solve this problem, use alligation medial. Change liters into mL 1 liter = 1000 mL 500 x 1.25 = 625 2500 x 0.81 = 2025 1500 x 1 = 1500 4500 4150 The new specific gravity is calculated as we calculated new concentration $= \dfrac{\Sigma (SG \times Q)}{\Sigma (Q)}$ Where SG = Specific gravity of mixture Q = Quantity or volume of liquid. $= \dfrac{4150}{4500} = 0.922$ Answer
Q238. 500 mL of an elixir with specific gravity 0.920 was mixed with 900 mL of glycerin having a specific gravity 1.250. Then 500 mL of Simple syrup with a specific gravity 1.300 was added to this mixture. Finally, water was added to make the total volume to 2 liters. What was the specific gravity of this product?	[the volume of water is obtained by subtracting the volume of the rest of ingredients from the total volume, = 2000 – (500+900+500) = 2000 – 1900 = 100 mL. Also specific gravity of water = 1.000] 0.920 x 500 = 460 1.250 x 900 = 1125 1.300 x 500 = 650 1.000 x 100 = 100 2000 2335 The new specific gravity = $\dfrac{\Sigma (SG \times Q)}{\Sigma (Q)}$ $\dfrac{2335}{2000} = 1.1675$ Answer.

| Q239. If we mix 200 mL of propylene glycol (Specific gravity 1.20) with 200 mL water, how many mL of additional propylene glycol should be added to change the specific gravity to 1.155 | Determine the specific gravity of the first mixture using alligation medial:

$200 \times 1.2 = 240$
$\underline{200 \times 1.0} = \underline{200}$
$400 \qquad\quad\; 440$

$$\frac{440}{400} = 1.10$$

Determine the required volume by alligation alternate:

$\begin{array}{lcl} 1.20 & & 0.055 \\ & 1.155 & \\ 1.10 & & 0.045 \end{array}$

The ratio of the required volume of propylene glycol to the first mixture $= 0.055:0.045 = 11:9$

400 mL = 9 parts. Calculate what is 11 parts:

$\dfrac{400}{x} = \dfrac{9}{11} \quad X = 488.9$ mL Answer.

Alternatively:
Let the volume of propylene glycol needed be V

$\begin{array}{llll} 200 & x & 1.2 & = 240 \\ 200 & x & 1.0 & = 200 \\ \underline{V} & x & 1.2 & = \underline{1.2V} \\ (200 + 200 + V) & & & (240 + 200 + 1.2V) \end{array}$

$$\frac{240 + 200 + 1.2V}{200 + 200 + V} = 1.155$$

$440 + 1.2V = 1.155(400 + V) = 462 + 1.155V$
$0.045V = 22$
$V = 488.9$ mL |

11.7.3 NOTES ON DILUTION OF ACIDS

An acid when undiluted is referred to as **concentrated acid**. The concentration of concentrated acids is expressed as percentage weight-in-weight (w/w). The concentration of Concentrated sulphuric acid for example is 96% **w/w.** This means that there are 96 grams of sulphuric acid in 100 g of the acid. When diluted, the concentration of the acid is expressed as percentage weight –in-volume. Thus 10%w/v sulphuric acid contains 10g of sulphuric acid in 100 mL of the acid.

You may be called upon to determine the volume of a concentrated acid required to prepare a desired quantity of a diluted acid. You may also be asked to calculate the concentration of a dilute acid when a given volume of water or any other liquid is added to the concentrated acid. In order to solve these problems, you will need to convert w/w to w/v or vice versa. Thus you need to know and apply the **specific gravity** of the concentrated acid to determine the volume required.

Q240. Calculate the volume of phosphoric acid required to prepare 500 mL bladder irrigation Solution containing 0.25% w/v phosphoric acid. Concentrated phosphoric acid is 85% w/w and has specific gravity 1.71	Strong phosphoric acid is 85% w/w. This means there are 85 f of pure phosphoric acid (100%) in 100grams of the acid. Bladder irrigation Solution is 0.25%w/v, which means there is 0.25 g in 100 mL of the solution. Find how many g of phosphoric acid are in 500 mL of the solution: = 0.25g x 5 = 1.25g Find how many grams of Conc.phosphoric acid shall contain 1.25 g: $\frac{100}{X} = \frac{85}{1.25}$ $X = 1.47\,g$ Calculate the volume of conc. phosphoric acid, given Sp Gravity = 1.71: $Volume = \frac{Weight}{specific\,Gravity} = \frac{1.47}{1.71} = 0.86\,mL$ Answer.
Q241. Concentrated sulphuric acid is 96% w/w, and has specific gravity 1.84. Calculate the volume of the concentrated acid required to prepare 2 liters of battery acid (33.5% w/v)	2 Liters (2000 mL) of dilute acid (33.5% w/v) are required. How many grams of sulphuric acid are required? $\frac{33.5}{100} \times 2000\,mL = 67g$ The conc. acid is 96%w/w, meaning there are 96 g in 100 g Calculate how many grams of the acid have 67 g sulphuric acid. $\frac{100}{X} = \frac{96}{67}$ $X = 69.8\,g$ To find the volume, $v = \frac{weight}{specific\,gravity} = \frac{69.8}{1.84} =$ = 64.65 mL Answer.

Q242. A pharmacy student diluted 200 mL of Concentrated hydrochloric acid (38% w/w, specific gravity 1.20) with enough water to make half a liter of dilute acid. Calculate the percent strength w/v of the dilute acid thus made.	38% w/w means there are 38 g of pure hydrochloric acid in 100g of conc. acid. Find the weight of 200 mL of the conc. acid if specific gravity is 1.20: $$weight = volume \times specific\ gravity$$ $$= 200 \times 1.20$$ $$= 240\ g$$ Calculate the weight of pure hydrochloric acid in 240 g of the 38% conc. acid: $$\frac{38}{100} \times 240 = 91.2\ g$$ Calculate the concentration of 91.2 g in 500 mL of dilute acid: $$\frac{91.2}{500} \times 100 = 18.24\%\ w/v\ \ Answer.$$

CHAPTER 12

EXPRESSION OF CONCENTRATION OF ELECTROLYTE SOLUTIONS:

MILLIEQUIVALENTS, MILLIMOLES AND MILLIOSMOLES

12.1 Introduction.

Compounds in solution are often referred to as either **electrolytes** or **non-electrolytes**. Electrolytes are compounds that in solution dissociate to varying degrees into "ions" which have an electrical charge. Examples: Sodium chloride (NaCl), Potassium chloride (KCl) and magnesium sulphate ($MgSO_4$). Non-electrolytes are compounds which do not dissociate in solution. Examples include dextrose and urea.

Electrolyte solutions or preparations are used for replacement of lost electrolytes (or electrolyte disturbances) as they occur in diarrhea, vomiting, excessive sweating and excessive urination. Electrolyte disturbance invariably leads to dehydration. Replacement of the lost electrolytes and fluids must be correctly balanced to just correct the loss and not to exceed the required amount.

As expressed in previous sections, concentration of pharmaceutical products can be expressed as mg/mL, mg%, g/L, g/100 mL or % strength, ratio strength, or parts per million. Electrolyte solutions are usually expressed as milliequivalents per liter (mEq/L), millimoles per liter mMol/L) or milliosmoles per liter(mOsmol/L). Pharmacists should understand and differentiate between these expressions so that he can explain and interconvert them when required to.

12.2 Milliequivalents:

Weight of a substance containing 1 Equivalent $= \dfrac{atomic\ (or\ oinic)weight\ (g)}{valence}$

Under normal operation this unit Equivalent is too large, and hence the unit that is commonly used is the **Milliequivalent**, which is $\dfrac{1}{1000}$ Equivalent weight, or just equivalent weight expressed in milligrams instead of gram:

Weight of the salt containing 1 Milliequivalent of an ion =

$$\dfrac{Molecular\ weight\ of\ the\ salt\ (expressed\ in\ mg)}{valence\ of\ the\ ion\ X\ Number\ of\ such\ ions\ in\ the\ molucule}$$

| Q243. Calculate the weight of sodium chloride that contains 1 Milliequivalent of Na^+ | Weight of the salt containing 1 mEq of an ion = $\dfrac{Molecular\ weight\ of\ the\ salt\ (in\ mg)}{valence\ of\ the\ ion\ X\ Number\ of\ such\ ions\ in\ the\ molucule}$

 Molecular weight of NaCl = 58.5 g
 Valence of $Na^+ = 1$
 There is only 1 ion in NaCl

 $= \dfrac{58.5\ mg}{1 \times 1} = 58.5mg$ |

Q244. How many grams of sodium chloride can supply 155 mEq of Na^+ per liter?	$58.5 \times 155 = 9067.5$ mg/L = 9.07 g/L The normal concentration of anions in plasma is 155 mEq. The answer of this question is the concentration of normal saline (0.9%)
Q245. Calculate the weight of Calcium chloride that contains 1 mEq of Cl^-	Mol wt of $CaCl_2$ = 147 Valence of Cl = 1 Number of Cl^- ion in $CaCl_2$ = 2 Weight of a substance containing 1 mEq = $$\frac{Molecular\ weight\ of\ the\ salt\ (in\ mg)}{valence\ of\ the\ ion \times Number\ of\ such\ ions\ in\ the\ molucule}$$ Weight containing 1 mEq of Cl^- = $\frac{147}{1 \times 2}$ = 73.5 mg
Q246. Calculate the weight of sodium phosphate ($Na_2HPO_4 \cdot 12H_2O$) that supplies 1 mEq of phosphate ion.	Mol wt of $Na_2HPO_4 \cdot 12H_2O$ is $(23 \times 2)+1+31+64+(12 \times 16)+(16 \times 12)$ = 358 Valence of HPO_4 = 2 Number of HPO_4 = 1 $$\frac{Molecular\ weight\ of\ the\ salt\ (in\ mg)}{valence\ of\ the\ ion \times Number\ of\ such\ ions\ in\ the\ molucule}$$ = $\frac{358}{2 \times 1}$ = 179 mg Answer

Table 1. ionic weight and Milliequivalent of common ions

Ion	Valence	Ionic weight	Milliequivalents (Ionic weight / valence)
Sodium (Na^+)	1	23	23
Potassium (K^+)	1	39	39
Calcium (Ca^{++})	2	40	20
Chloride (Cl^-)	1	35.5	35.5
Bicarbonate (HCO_3^-)	1	61	61
Phosphate (HPO_4^{2-})	2	96	48
Phosphate ($H_2PO_4^-$)	1	97	97
Citrate ($C_6H_5O_7^{3-}$)	3	189	63

Concentration of electrolytes infusions is usually expressed as Milliequivalent per liter (mEq/L). This expression indicates absolute number of particles which expresses the actual chemical combining power of electrolytes. When mEq are used, the relationship between ions is accurately portrayed and one can see that the number of anions = number of cations. When the concentration is expressed in terms of actual weights the relationship between cations and anions cannot be deciphered.

The expression mEq/L depends on the number of particles in the solution and the total number of ionic charges, that is the valence of the ion, and that makes the measurement more meaningful. Table 2 compares the values expressed as mg and the same values expressed in mEq: The table shows a clear balance between anions and cations, both of which are 155. But when the values are expressed as grams, this balance is not seen and actually it appears as if there are more cations than anions.

Table 2. Average Normal of Blood Plasma.

	MEq/L	mg /100mL
Cations:		
Na^+	142	327
K^+	5	20
Mg^{++}	3	4
Ca^{++}	5	10
Total	155	361
Anions		
HCO_3^-	27	165
Cl^-	103	366
HPO_4^-	2	10
SO_4^-	1	5
Organic acids	6	?
Proteins	16	7100
Total	155	7646

Having understood what an equivalent is, you should now be able to convert the concentration of electrolytes expressed as Milliequivalent per unit volume to weight per unit volume or percent strength and vice versa.

Q247. Calculate the concentration in g/L of a solution containing 2 mEq of potassium chloride per mL.	Molecular weight of potassium chloride (KCl) = 74.5
	Milliequivalent of KCl = $\frac{74.5}{1 \times 1}$ = 74.5mg
	2 Milliequivalent per mL = 2 x 74.5 = 149 mg /mL
	                               = 149000mg/L
	                               = 149 g/L
	
	NOTE THAT To convert mEq/mL to mg/mL :
	
	mg/mL = (mEq per mL)X (Number of mg containing 1 mEq)
	
	      = 2 X 74.5
	      = 149 mg/mL

Q248. Convert 120mEq/L of ammonium chloride to percent w/v concentration	Molecular weight of NH_4Cl = 53.5 Equivalent weight of NH_4Cl = 53.5 (valence = 1, Number of molecules = 1) 1 Eq of NH_4Cl = 53.5 g therefore 1 mEq = 53.5 mg 120 mEq = 53.5 mg x 120 = 6420 mg = 6.420 g /L

	6.420 g/L = 0.642 g/100 mL = 0.642% Answer
	To convert meEq/L to % w/v:
	$\%w/v = \dfrac{(mEq\ per\ L) \times (Number\ of\ grams\ containing\ 1\ mEq)}{10}$
	$mEq/mL = \dfrac{\%\frac{w}{v} \times 10}{Number\ of\ grams\ containing\ 1\ mEq}$
Q249. The label of on injection ampule reads "2.98 g/10 mL" potassium chloride. Express this concentration as "mEq/mL"	Molecular weight of potassium chloride = 74.5 1 Milliequivalent of KCl = 74.5 mg Convert 2.98 g/10 mL to mEq/10 mL: 2.98 g = 2980 mg = $\dfrac{2980}{74.5}$ mEq = 40 mEq/10 mL The concentration = 4 mEq/mL Answer To convert mg/mL to mEq/mL: $mEq/mL = \dfrac{mg\ per\ mL}{number\ of\ mg\ containing\ 1\ mEq}$
Q250. A solution contains 25 mg% of Ca^{++} ions. What is this concentration in mEq/mL? What the concentration in mg/L?	25 mg% = 25 mg in 100 mL Ionic weight Ca^{++} = 40 Weight containing 1 mEq of Ca^{++} = $\dfrac{40}{1 \times 2}$ (Valence of Ca = 2) = 20 mg Number of mEq in 100 mL = $\dfrac{25\ mg}{20\ mg}$ = 1.25 mEq/100mL = 0.0125 mEq/mL Answer. = 0.0125 × 1000 mEq/L = 125 mEq/L Answer.
Q251. How many mL of 3%w/v solution of ammonium chloride (NH_4Cl – Mol wt = 53.5) should be intravenously administered to a patient to provide 50 mEq?	3% = 3 g in 100 mL 1 mEq of NH_4Cl = 53.5 mg 50 mEq = 53.5 × 50 = 2675 mg = 2.675 g If 3g are in 100 mL, how many mL contain 2.675 g? $\dfrac{3\ g}{2.675\ g} = \dfrac{100\ ml}{X\ mL}$ X = 89.2 mL Answer
Q252. Express 154 mEq/L of sodium chloride solution as mg%	Molecular weight of NaCl = 58.5 (23 + 35.5) 1 mEq of NaCl = $\dfrac{Mol\ wt}{valence}$ = $\dfrac{58.5}{1}$ = 58.5 mg 154 mEq = 154 × 58.5 g = 9009 mg The solution has 9009mg /L = 900.9 mg/100 mL = 901 mg% Answer.

Q253. A 500 mL bottle of Ammonium chloride is labeled as 21.4 mg/mL. How many mEq of ammonium chloride are in the full bottle of the solution? (Mol Wt of NH_4Cl = 53.5).	$1\ mEq\ of\ NH_4Cl = 53.5\ mg$ Total amount of NH_4Cl in 500 mL = 21.4 mg/mL x 500 mL = 10700 mg Total number of $mEq = \frac{10700mg}{53.5mg} = 200\ mEq$ Answer { concentration = 200 mEq/500mL or 0.4 mEq/mL}
Q254. ℞: Methicillin Na 1g qid x 5/7 How many mEq of sodium will the patient receive in total? (Mol Wt of methicillin, $C_{17}H_{19}NaO_6S.H_2O$ = 420)	Since the valence of Na = 1, and there is only 1 Na in the molecular formula, 1 mEq of methicillin = 420 mg Total dose = 1 g x 4 per day x 5 days = 20 g = 20,000 mg Total number of $mEq = \frac{20000mg}{420\ mg} = 47.6\ mEq$ Answer
Q255. How many mEq are in 20g magnesium sulphate $(MgSO_4)$?	Molecular weight of $MgSO_4$ = 24+32+(4x16)= 120 $$\frac{Molecular\ weight\ of\ the\ salt\ (in\ mg)}{valence\ of\ the\ ion\ X\ Number\ of\ such\ ions\ in\ the\ molucule}$$ Valence Mg = 2, Number of Mg ions in the molecule = 1 $1\ mEq\ of\ MgSO_4 = \frac{120}{2x1} = 60$ There are 20 g of Magnesium sulphate = 20,000 mg 20000 mg of $MgSO_4 = \frac{20,000}{60} = 333.3\ mEq$ Answer OR $\frac{60mg}{20,000mg} = \frac{1mEq}{X\ mEq}$ X = 333.3 mg

Q256.
℞:
Potassium acetate   5 g ($C_2H_3KO_2$ Mol wt = 98)
Potassium bicarbonate 5 g ($KHCO_3$ Mol wt = 100)
Potassium citrate   5 g ($C_6H_5K_3O_7.H_2O$ Mol wt = 324)
Water   Ad 50 mL
Sig: 1 tsp 0D 3/7

How many mEq of potassium are in each dose?
  To solve this problem, consider each salt separately.
  Each dose = 1 teaspoonful = 5 mL
  If there are 5 g in 50 mL, then there is 0.5 g in 5 mL= 500mg

  Potassium acetate Mol wt = 98,
    K has valence 1 and there is 1 ion of K, thus 1 mEq = 98 mg
    The number of mEq in 500 mL = $\frac{1mEq}{XmEq} = \frac{98mg}{500mg}$ x = 5.1 mEq
    Potassium bicarbonate Mol wt = 100
    K has valence 1 and there is only 1 ion of K, thus mEq = 100 mg

The number of mEq in 500 mL : $\frac{1mEq}{xmEq} = \frac{100}{500}$ $X = 5\ mEq$

Potassium citrate Mol wt = 324

K valence = 1, there 3 K ions in the molecule, thus 1 mEq = $\frac{324}{1 \times 3}$ = 106 mg

The number of mEq in 500 mg: $\frac{1mEq}{xmEq} = \frac{106}{500}$ $x = 4.7\ mEq$

Total number of mEq of potassium = 5.1+5+4.7= 14.8 mEq Answer.

Q257. ℞: NH₄Cl 36mg/Kg body wt Mol wt of NH₄Cl = 53.5 Ammonium chloride solution is available as 500mEq/L. How many mL of the sterile solution should be administered to 65 kg person to provide the required dose?	Total amount of ammonium chloride required 　　　　= 36 mg/kg x 65 kg 　　　　= 2340 mg 1 mEq of NH₄Cl = 53.5 Total number of mEq required: $\frac{1mEq}{X} = \frac{53.5mg}{2340mg}$ $x = 43.7\ mEq$ But there are 500 mEq per liter or per 1000 mL. How many mL will provide 43.7 mEq? $\frac{1000mL}{X} = \frac{500mEq}{43.7mEq}$ $X = 87.4\ mL$ Answer.
Q258. 20 mL of a 5 mEq per mL solution of potassium chloride (Mol wt 74.5) were diluted with water to one liter. What is the percent strength of the resulting solution? with water	Total number of mEq in 20 mL = 5 mEq/mL x 20 mL = 100 mEq 1 mEq of KCl = 74.5mg 100 mEq = 74.5x 100 = 7450 mg After dilution, there are 7450 mg in 1 L = 7.450g in 1000 mL 　　　　　　　　　　　　= 0.745 g in 100 mL 　　　　　　　　　　　　= 0.745%w.v
Q259. 500 mL sodium chloride solution was diluted to 12.5 liters with water. The concentration of the diluted solution was 1.17% w/v. Calculate the concentration of the original solution in percent strength and in mEq/mL	In the final solution (1.17%), there are 1.17 g in 100 mL The total solution available = 12.5 L = 12500 mL The total amount of sodium chloride in the whole diluted solution: $\frac{1.17g}{Xg} = \frac{100mL}{12500mL}$ $x= 146.25g$ This amount was originally in 500 mL The concentration of the original solution = 146.25g/500mL To find the percent strength determine how much is in 100 mL 　　　　　　　　　　　　= $146.25 \times \frac{100}{500}$g/100 mL 　　　　　　　　　　　　= 29.25% w/answer. The concentration 29.25% means There are 29.25g in 100 mL 　　　　　　　　Or there are 29250mg in 100 mL 　　　　Or there are 292.5 mg in 1 mL 1 mEq of sodium chloride = 58.5 mg 292.5 mg/mL = $\frac{292.5}{58.5}$mEq/mL = 5 mEq/mL Answer.

Q260. How many grams of sodium bicarbonate (NaHCO₃ Mol wt = 84) should be used to prepare 500 mL of solution having a concentration of 1.8 mEq/2 mL solution?	The final concentration has 1.8 mEq per 2 mL. We find how much is in 500 mL $\frac{1.8mEq}{X} = \frac{2mL}{500mL}$ X = 450 mEq 1 mEq of NaHCO₃ = 84 mg 450 mEq = 84 x 450 = 37800 mg = 37.8 g Answer.

12.3 MILLIMOLES

In SI units, the unit of a chemical quantity is the **mole** instead of **Equivalent and Milliequivalent**. The units of biochemical composition of the body and concentration of infusion fluids have changed from the Milliequivalent to the mole notation.

1 Mole = amount of substance containing as many elementary units (atoms, molecules, ions etc.) as there are atoms in 12 g of carbon isotope ^{12}C. (this number of elementary units is Avogadro's Number = 6.023×10^{23})

However, the composition of biochemical entities in the body are usually in small quantities and hence mole unit is too large. Therefore, its sub unit, the Millimole is more often used.

The mole of a **molecule** is the same as its **gram molecular weight**.

The weight of a substance containing 1 Millimole (mmol) = $\frac{gram\ molecular\ weight\ (g)}{1000}$

Or = *gram molecular wt (expressed in mg)*

Dextrose has a molecular weight of 180 g.

Weight of dextrose containing 1 mmol = 180 mg.

A mole of an **ion** is its **ionic weight**. However, the number of moles of an ion of a salt in a solution depends on the **number** of each ion in the molecule of the salt:

> One mole of Sodium Chloride (NaCl) provides 1 mole of sodium (Na^+) ions and one mole of Chloride (Cl^-) ions. The molecular weight of sodium chloride provides one mole of Na^+ and one mole of Cl^-

> One mole of calcium chloride (Ca Cl₂) has one Ca^{++} and two Cl^- and hence the molecular weight of calcium chloride provides 1 mole Ca^{++} and 2 moles Cl^-

Therefore the quantity of salt, in milligrams, containing mmol of a particular ion can be found by dividing the molecular weight of the salt by the number of the ions contained in the salt.

$$1\ mmol\ of\ an\ ion = \frac{M.Wt\ (mg)}{Number\ of\ such\ ions\ in\ the\ molecule}$$

Table 5: weights of salts containing 1 mmol of an ion

Salt	Ion	Quantity of salt (in mg) containing 1 mmol
NaCl	Na^+	Mol wt ÷ 1 = 58.5
	Cl^-	Mol wt ÷ 1 = 58.5
$CaCl_2$	Ca^{++}	Mol wt ÷ 1 = 147
	Cl^-	Mol wt ÷ 2 = 73.5
Na_2HPO_4	Na^+	Mol wt ÷ 2 = 179
	HPO_4^{2-}	Mol wt ÷ 1 = 258
NaH_2PO_4	Na^+	Mol wt ÷ 1 = 156
	$H_2PO_4^-$	Mol wt ÷ 1 = 156
$CH_3COONa.3H_2O$	CH_3COO^-	Mol wt ÷ 1 = 136

mg per liter = (number of mg of a salt containing 1 mmol) X (number of mmol per liter)

Q261. Calculate how much of potassium chloride (Mol wt 74.5), Magnesium chloride (Mol Wt 203); Calcium Chloride (Mol wt 147) and sodium chloride (Mol wt 58.5) are required to provide the following electrolyte in 1 liter of water?
 	
Na^+ 60 mmol
K^+ 5 mmol
Mg^{++} 4 mmol
Ca^{++} 4 mmol
Cl^- 81 mmol
	5 mmol of K^+ are provided by KCl 74.5 mg x 5 = 0.373 g
	   (it also provides 5 mmol of Chloride)
	4 mmol of Mg^{++} provided by $MgCl_2$ 203 mg x 4 = 0.812 g
	   (it also provides 2 x4 mmol of chloride)
	4 mmol of Ca^{++} are provided by $CaCl_2$ 4 x 147 mg = 0.588g
	   (it also provides 2x4 mmol of Chloride)
	60 mmol of Na^+ are provided by 60 x 58.5 mg = 3.510 g
	   (it also provides 60 mmol of Chloride)

Q262. DNS infusion contains 4.3% w/v dextrose and 0.18% w/v sodium chloride. How many Millimole of each component are in one liter of the infusion?	4.3% and 0.18% means 4.3 g in 100 mL and 0.18g in 100 mL respectively.
	Thus in 1 Liter there are 43 g of dextrose = 43000 mg
	and 1.8 g of sodium chloride = 1800 mg.
	Molecular weight of dextrose = 180
	    Amount containing 1 mmol dextrose = 180 mg
	Molecular weight of Sodium chloride = 58.5
	    Amount containing 1 mmol NaCl = 58.5 mg

	$Mmol\ od\ dextrose = \frac{43,000\ mg}{180} = 238.9\ mmol$ Answer
	$Mmol\ of\ NaCl = \frac{1800}{58.5} = 30.8\ mmol$ Answer
Q263. Calculate the number of mmol of calcium and chloride ions in one liter of 0.029 % w/v solution of Calcium chloride	*0.029% means 0.029g in 100 mL. Therefore in 1 liter(1000 mL) there are 0.29 g or 290 mg of calcium chloride.* *Molecular weight of calcium chloride = 147* *1 mmol of $CaCl_2$ = 147 mg . Calculate how many mmol are in 290 mg:* $\frac{1\ mmol}{X\ mmol} = \frac{147}{290}$ $X = 2\ mmol$ *But each mole of $CaCl_2$ provides one mole of calcium and 2 moles of chloride ions. Therefore 1 liter contains* *2 mmols of Ca^{++} and 4mmol of Cl^- Answer.*

12.4 MILLIOSMOLES

In chemistry, the **osmole** (**Osm** or **osmol**) is a non-SI unit of measurement that defines the number of moles of a chemical compound that contribute to a solution's osmotic pressure. The term comes from the phenomenon of osmosis, and is typically used for osmotically-active solutions. An osmole is an amount of substance containing Avogadro's number of osmotically active particles.

Osmotic pressure is very important in physiology. Biological processes involve diffusion of solutes and transfer of fluids through semi-permeable membranes. Thus the knowledge of osmolar concentrations of parenteral fluids is paramount. Indeed sometimes the concentrations of body fluids and fluid replacement solutions are expressed in osmoles, a unit that reflects osmotic activities.

A solution of dextrose containing 1 mmol per kg of water has an osmolality of 1 mosmL/kg. Likewise, a solution of 1 mol/L NaCl corresponds to an osmolarity of 2 osmol/L. The NaCl salt particle dissociates fully in water to become two separate particles: an Na^+ ion and a Cl^- ion. Therefore, each mole of NaCl becomes two osmoles in solution, one mole of Na^+ and one mole of Cl^-. Similarly, a solution of 1 mol/L $CaCl_2$, gives a solution of 3 osmol/L (Ca^{2+} and 2 Cl^-).

Osmotic pressure is proportional to total number of particles in the solution. The milliosmole = 1 mmol for non-electrolytes and increase with the degree of dissociation. Assuming complete dissociation**,

1mmol sodium chloride (NaCl)   = 2 mOsmol
1mmol Calcium chloride ($CaCl_2$)   = 3 mOsmol
1 mmol Sodium citrate ($Na_3C_6H_5O_7$) = 4 mOsmol

** This is only true in dilute solutions. In concentrated solutions, osmolality is affected by particle interaction and a correction factor (the osmolar coefficient which has been determined should be used)

Like for the unit mole, Osmol is a large unit. In practice a mOsmol is used which is 1000th of the Osmol

$$mOsmol = \frac{wt\ of\ substance\ \left(\frac{g}{L}\right)}{Mol\ wt\ of\ the\ substance} X\ Number\ of\ species\ x\ 1000$$

Q264. Express 0.9% Sodium Chloride in mOsmol/L	$mOsmol =$ $\frac{wt\ of\ substance\ \left(\frac{g}{L}\right)}{Mol\ wt\ of\ the\ substance} X\ Number\ of\ species\ x\ 1000$ $= \frac{9\left(\frac{g}{L}\right)}{58.5g} X\ 2\ X\ 1000 = 308\ mOsmol/L$
Q265. Express 4.5% dextrose in mOsmol/L	Molecular weight of dextrose = 180 5% dextrose solution contains 5 g in 100 mL of solution = 5000 mg/100 mL = 50000 mg/L $mOsmols = \frac{wt\ of\ substance\ (mg)}{mol\ wt}\ x\ \#\ species$ = 50000 ÷ 180 = 278 m Osmol/L Answer
Q266. What is the osmolality of 8.4% NH_4HCO_3?	Mol.wt of NH_4HCO_3 is 79 8.4% = 8.4 g / 100 mL = 84g/L $Osmolarity = \frac{84}{79} =$ 1.06 $Osmol/L$
Q267. Calculate the number of a) mmol b) mEq c) mOsmol present in 294 mL of 10% solution of Calcium chloride ($CaCl_2.2H_2O$, Mol wt = 147)	10% = 10g per 100 mL Amount in 294 mL: $\frac{10}{x} = \frac{100mL}{294mL}$ $X = 29.4\ g = 29400\ mg$ $Mmol = \frac{available\ wt}{Mol\ wt} = \frac{29400}{147} = 200\ mmol\ Answer$ $mEq = \frac{available\ wt}{Mol\ wt} x\ Valence = \frac{29000}{147} x\ 2 = 400\ mEq\ Ans.$ $mOsmol = \frac{available\ wt}{Mol\ wt}\ x\ Number\ of\ species$ $= \frac{29000}{147} x\ 3 = 600\ mEq/L\ Answer$

CHAPTER 13

ISOTONIC SOLUTIONS

13.1 Introduction

Movement of fluids from one body compartment to another, such as for example from blood in blood vessels to body cells, or from adipose (or fatty) tissues to the space between body cells (interstitial space) is via a phenomenon known as osmosis. The body compartments are separated by semi-permeable membrane. Specifically, **Osmosis** is movement of fluid from dilute solution to a more concentrated solution when the two solutions are separated by a semi-permeable membrane. This movement is dependent on **osmotic pressure** as the driving force. Osmotic pressure is dependent on the number of particles present in the solution.

Substances which dissociate in solution (breaking into separate particles) such as ionic substances are called **electrolytes**. Sodium chloride for example dissociates into sodium ions (Na^+) and Chloride ions (Cl^-). The degree to which electrolyte dissociate will dictate the number of particles available and these in turn will determine the osmotic pressure. Thus for electrolytes, osmotic pressure and hence osmosis depends both on concentration of the electrolyte and its degree of dissociation.

Solutions which have the same osmotic pressure are known as **iso-osmotic solutions.** When separated by a semi-permeable membrane, iso-osmotic solutions do not exhibit any overall movement of fluid in any direction. The fluids are said to be in equilibrium, the fluid moving equally in both direction of the semi-permeable membrane. Solutions with same osmotic pressure as body fluid are known as **isotonic solutions**. **Isotonicity** is important in eye and nasal preparations, irrigation fluids, parenteral and enema preparations. If these preparations are not isotonic with body fluids, they tend to cause irritation and pain. The terms **hypotonic** and **hypertonic solutions** refer to solutions with lower and higher osmotic pressure respectively and both are known also as **paratonic solutions**.

13.2 Using colligative properties to determine isotonic concentrations:

For **non-electrolytes**, osmosis is determined by the number of molecules and therefore their concentrations. Dextrose and boric acid are examples of non-electrolytes. Such molecules do not dissociate.

Properties that depend on the number of particles available in a given solvent or fluid such as osmosis (or osmotic pressure) are called **colligative properties**. Other colligative properties apart from osmosis include **vapor pressure lowering, boiling point elevation and freezing point depression.**

Theoretically one can use any of the colligative properties to calculate the amount of a substance needed to attain isotonicity, but osmotic pressure and freezing point depression are used because they are is simple to determine and hence are practical.

Important facts: it is important to learn these facts by heart as they are handy when doing calculations involving isotonicity.

1. the freezing point of blood serum, , tears, saliva and lachrymal fluid = -0.52°C
2. The freezing point of 1 gram-molecular weight of any non-dissociating substance in 1L (1000mL) = -1.86°C
3. 0.3 mole in 1L of any solution is isotonic
4. A solution of 9 g sodium chloride in 1 Liter of water or 0.9% w/v is isotonic with body fluids
5. Blood plasma and lachrymal fluid exert osmotic pressure of 6.7 atmospheres per liter.

Boric acid has molecular weight 61.8. This is 1 gram-molecular weight. From the facts above, the freezing point of 61.8g boric acid in 1L = -1.86°C. We can therefore find the amount of boric acid in a solution that is isotonic with blood plasma, by calculating the concentration of boric acid that freezes at the same temperature as plasma(-0.52°C).

If you are dealing with electrolytes do not forget to consider that electrolytes dissociate and therefore you may have more particles than would be expected from non-electrolytes. For example, sodium chloride in a weak solution is about 80% dissociated. This means for every 100 molecules of sodium chloride there are 80 ions of Na^-, 80 ions of Cl^- and 20 molecules of NaCl making a total number of particles 180 OR this can be expressed as 100 molecules of NaCl yield 1.8 times more particles than the same number of non-dissociating substance or non-electrolyte. The value 1.8 is the **dissociation constant** of sodium chloride and should be included in the calculation for isotonicity.

Q268. A solution of dextrose (Mol wt 180) contains 45g in 500 mL. Calculate the freezing point of the solution.	1 gram molecular weight of a substance freezes at -1.86°C Thus 180 g of dextrose in 1 L of water freezes at 1.86°C
	The dextrose solution contains 45 g in 500 mL. It will therefore contain 90 g in 1 liter.
	The freezing point of dextrose solution (90g/1000 mL) is:
	$\frac{180}{90} = \frac{1.86}{X}$ $X = 0.93$ = -0.93°C Answer
Q269. Molecular weight of boric acid is 61.8. Calculate the concentration of boric acid that is isotonic with blood plasma	1 gram Mol wt in one liter freezes at -1.86°C 61.8 g/L freezes at -1.86°C. The concentration of boric acid that is isotonic with blood plasma freezes at -0.52°C Let us find the concentration of boric acid that freezes at – 0.52°C
	$\frac{61.8g}{Xg} = \frac{1.86°C}{0.52°C}$ $X = 17.3g/L$ Answer = 1.73% w/v Answer
Q270. Calculate the concentration of sodium chloride that is isotonic with lachrymal fluids (Mol wt of NaCl is 58.5)	58.5 g of sodium chloride freezes at -1.86°C x 1.8 because NaCl dissociates by 1.8. There are 1.8 times as many particles as there are in a non-dissociating substance. Let us find the concentration of NaCl that is

	isotonic with lachrymal fluid (-0.52°C) $$\frac{58.5g}{X} = \frac{1.86°C \times 1.8}{0.52°C} \quad X = 9.09 g/L$$ $= 0.91\% w/v$ Answer

General formula for calculation of concentration of isotonic fluid:

$$G \text{ of solute per Liter of an isotonic solution} = \frac{0.52 \times Molecular\ weight}{1.86 \times dissociation\ factor}$$

$$= 0.28 \times \frac{molecular\ weight}{dissociation\ factor}$$

$$= 0.28 \times \frac{M}{i} \quad \text{Where M = Molecular weight}$$
$$\quad i = \text{dissociation factor}$$

Q271. Calculate the concentration of procaine hydrochloride (Mol Wt 273, dissociation factor = 1.8) that is isotonic with blood plasma	$0.28 \times \frac{273}{1.8} = 42.47\ g/L = 4.2\% w/v$ Answer.
Q272. Zinc sulphate (ZnSO$_4$), a 2-ion electrolyte is said to dissociate by 40%. Calculate its dissociation factor	This is a 2-ion electrolyte that dissociates 40% Therefore 100 particles of zinc sulphate shall dissociate to give 40 particles of Zn^{++}, 40 particles of SO_4 and 60 particles of $ZnSO_4$, a total of 140 particles. Thus 100 molecule produce 140 particles The dissociation factor is 1.4. Answer
Q273. Zinc chloride, ZnCl$_2$ is a 3-ion electrolyte with 80% dissociation. Calculate its dissociation factor	100 particles of will dissociate to give 80 particles of Zn^{++}, 80 x2 = 160 particles of Cl^- and 20 particles of $ZnCl_2$ 100 particles produce A total of 260 particles. The dissociation factor = 2.6 Answer.
Q274. Sodium chloride is a 2-ion electrolyte, dissociating 90% in solution. Calculate its dissociation factor	100 particles dissociate to give 90 particles of Na^+; 90 particles of Cl^- and 10 particles of NaCl that is a total of 190 particles. Thus the dissociation constant = 1.9 Answer..

Dissociation factors (i) of many medicinal substances have not been experimentally determined. If the dissociation factor has not been provided you can estimate it by applying the following rules.

1. If better information is not available, use the following values.
   a. If a substance dissociates into 2 ions   i = 1.8
   b. If a substance dissociates into 3 ions   i = 2.6
   c. If a substance dissociates into 4 ions   i = 3.4
   d. If a substance dissociates into 5 ions   i = 4.2
   e. non electrolytes i = 1

13 3. Making Isotonic Solutions, Use of Sodium Chloride equivalents.

Most medicinal solutions are hypotonic. The therapeutic concentrations of injectable is usually lower than that of body fluids. If they were to be injected as such, they would cause pain or irritation, a situation that would discomfort users, the patients. In order to make them isotonic, an inert substance (which does not cause any ill effect neither on the medicine nor to the user)is added to the solution. The concentration of the added substance is calculated so as to add the deficient fraction to achieve the exact isotonic concentration with the active ingredient.

For example we know that 0.9% sodium chloride solution is isotonic with blood plasma. Suppose you were given a 0.45% sodium chloride solution and you were asked to make it isotonic with blood plasma, just add enough to make 0.9%. In this case if you were give 100 mL of a 0.45% NaCl, just add another 0.45 g of NaCl and you get the required isotonic concentration, 0.9%. But if we had 1% solution of atropine sulphate we have to calculate how much sodium chloride this 1% solution of atropine sulphate represents, and therefore in order to make it isotonic how much more sodium chloride is needed, to make an effect of 09% NaCl. This brings us to the idea of **Sodium Chloride Equivalent.**

Sodium chloride equivalent =Number of grams of sodium chloride having the same tonicity (or tonic effect) as 1 gram of the substance.

| Q275. Calculate the amount of sodium chloride (Mol wt 58.5, dissociation constant =1.8) that have the same tonic effect as 1 gram of boric acid (Mol wt =61.8, dissociation constant = 1)

• [the answer is the sodium chloride equivalent of boric acid] | The tonic effect of 1 g Mol wt of boric acid is the same as 1 g Mol wt X 1.8 of sodium chloride.
$$61.8 \equiv 58.5/1.8$$

Let us find out the tonic effect of 1 g of boric acid is equivalent to how many grams of sodium chloride:
$$1\,g \equiv ?\,g$$
$$\frac{61.8}{1} = \frac{\frac{58.5}{1.8}}{X}$$
$$\frac{61.8}{1} = \frac{32.5}{X}$$

$$X = 0.52\,g$$

This means 1 g of boric acid has the same tonic effect as 0.52 g sodium chloride. **The sodium chloride equivalent of boric acid is 0.52**

1 g /100mL of boric acid is the same as having 0.52g/100mL sodium chloride. So if you want to make 100 mL of 1% boric acid isotonic, you need to add 0.9-0.52=0.38 g of sodium chloride. |

Q276. Calculate how much sodium chloride (Mol wt 58.5, I = 1.8) is represented by 1g atropine sulphate (mol.wt. 695, i= 2.6) • [the answer is sodium chloride equivalent of atropine sulphate]	The tonic effect of $\frac{695g}{2.6}$ atropine sulphate is the same as $\frac{58.5g}{1.8}$ of sodium chloride $\frac{695}{2.6} \equiv \frac{58.5}{1.8}$ $267.3 \equiv 32.5$ $1g \equiv ?$ $\frac{263}{1} = \frac{32.5}{X}$ X= 0.12g Answer Therefore 1 gram of atropine sulphate has the same tonic effect as 0.12 g sodium chloride. **The sodium chloride equivalent of atropine sulphate is 0.12**
Sodium chloride equivalent of a substance $= M_{NaCl}/\, i_{NaCl}$ $M_{substance}/\, I$ substance **Where M_{NaCl}= Mol wt of NaCl** **i_{NaCl} = Dissociation constant of NaCl** **$M_{substance}$= Mol wt of the substance** **$i_{substance}$ = Dissociation constant of the substance** $\frac{Molecular\ weight\ of\ NaCl}{dissociation\ constant\ of\ NaCl} \times \frac{Dissociation\ constant\ of\ the\ substance}{Molecular\ weight\ of\ the\ substance}$ $\frac{58.5}{1.8} X \frac{i}{M} = \frac{32.5\, i}{M}$ Where i is dissociation constant of a substance M is its molecular weight.	
Q277. Calculate the sodium chloride equivalent of papaverine hydrochloride (Mol wt = 376, dissociation constant = 1.8)	Sodium chloride equivalent = $\frac{32.5\, i}{M}$ M= 376, i = 1.8 Sodium chloride equivalent = $\frac{32.5 \times 1.8}{376} = 0.156$ or approx 0.16 Answer.
Q278. Procaine hydrochloride is a two-ion molecule, Mol wt = 273. What is the sodium chloride equivalent of procaine HCl?	Sodium chloride equivalent = $\frac{32.5\, i}{M}$ M = 276 Being a two-ion molecule and i is not given we assume i = 1.8 Sodium chloride equivalent = $\frac{32.5}{276} x 1.8 = 0.21$

Sodium chloride equivalents of many substances used in pharmaceutical preparations have been determined and are listed in table 4. Use this table as a reference to obtain these values when needed.

13.4 CALCULATIONS INVOLVING DETERMINATION OF ISOTONIC CONCENTRATIONS

1. Use sodium Chloride equivalents.

In order to calculate the amount of tonic agent required to make a give solution isotonic the following rules are followed:

I. Calculate the amount in g of sodium chloride represented by the ingredients in the prescription
Apply the knowledge of Sodium chloride equivalent and multiply the number of grams of each substance by its sodium chloride equivalent to find the amount of NaCl represented. Add the values obtained in all ingredients
$\sum$ (weight in grams x e)
II. Calculate the amount in grams of sodium chloride alone that would be contained in the isotonic solution of the volume specified in the prescription (This is the amount of sodium chloride in 0.9% solution. For example for 50 mL of 0.9% sodium chloride solution, we need 0.45 g in 50 mL to make it 0.9%)
III. Subtract the amount of sodium chloride represented by the ingredients in the prescription (I) from the amount of sodium chloride in (II). The answer is the amount of sodium chloride to be added to the solution.
IV. If you are using substances other than sodium chloride e.g. dextrose, sodium nitrate, boric acid or lactose, divide the amount of sodium chloride in (III) by the sodium chloride equivalent (e) of the substance to be used.

| Q279. Calculate how much sodium chloride is required in this prescription to make the following formular for the Eye isotonic with blood plasma:

Pilocarpine nitrate   0.3g
Sodium chloride   qs
Purified water ad   30mL | The formula is to make 30 mL of a solution containing 0.3 g pilocarpine nitrate. This solution is hypotonic. We need to add sodium chloride to make isotonic

Step i: calculate the equivalent amount of NaCl represented by each ingredient by multiplying its amount with its sodium chloride equivalent: i) 0.22 x 0.3 = 0.066
0.3 g of pilocarpineNO₃ have same tonicity as 0.066 g NaCl

Step ii: If we wanted to make 30mL of isotonic NaCl solution (0.9%)how much NaCl would we need?
$$ii) \ 30 \times \frac{0.9}{100} = 0.27$$
We need 0.27 g of NaCl to make 30mL of isotonic solution

Step iii: Subtract the amount of sodium chloride represented by the ingredients in the prescription (step i) from the amount of sodium chloride in (step ii).
$$iii) \ 0.27 - 0.066 = 0.204$$

The amount of sodium chloride required = 0.204g. |

Q280. How many grams of sodium chloride would be required to be added to the following Eye formular to make it isotonic with blood plasma?
 	
℞:
Scopolamine HBr   1/3 %
Dipivefrin HCl   ½ %
Sodium Chloride   q.s.
Purified water   ad   60 mL
	Referring in table 4,
	    sodium chloride equivalent of scopolamine = 0.13
	    Sodium chloride equivalent of Dipivefrin = 0.15
	
	Scopolamine is 1/3% which means 0.33 g in 100 mL solution
	    $= 0.33 \times \frac{60}{100}$ in 60 mL = 0.198 g
	Dipivefrin is ½ % which means 0.5 g in 100 mL
	    $= 0.5 \times \frac{60}{100} =$ in 60 mL = 0.5 g
	Step 1: equivalence of scopolamine = 0.198 x 0.13 = 0.0257
	Equivalence of Dipivefrine = 0.5 x 0.15 = 0.075
	    TOTAL 0.132
	Step 2: How much NaCl would be required in 60 mL
	                              $60 \times \frac{0.9}{100}$ = 0.54 g
	
	Step 3: = (step 2)-(step 1)
	          = 0.54- 0.132
	          = 0.408 g Answer

Q281. How much potassium nitrate is needed to make 30 mL of 0.5% silver nitrate isotonic with lachrymal fluid?	Silver nitrate in incompatible with sodium chloride. The latter cannot therefore be used to adjust isotonicity for silver nitrate solution. Potassium nitrate is used instead.
	
	From the reference table,
	    sodium chloride equivalent of potassium nitrate = 0.58
	    sodium chloride equivalent of silver nitrate = 0.34
	
	Amount of silver nitrate required in the prescription
	                                            = 0.5% x 30 mL = 0.15 g
	Step 1: 0.34 x 0.15 = 0.051g (NaCl represented by 0.15 g AgNO$_3$)
	Step 2: 30mL x 0.9% = 0.27 g (NaCl required to make 30 mL isotonic)
	Step 3: 0.27 - 0.051 = 0.219 g (amount of NaCl that would be required to make the solution isotonic)
	Step iv: Since NaCl and AgNo3 are incompatible, we are using potassium nitrate instead of sodium chloride. We obtain the
	    amount of KNO$_3$ required by dividing the amount of NaCl required by the sodium chloride equivalent of KNO$_3$
	    0.219 ÷ 0.58 = 0.38g of KNO$_3$

Q282
Phenacaine HCl   1%
Chlorbutanol   0.5%
Boric acid   q.s.
Purified water   ad   60 mL
 	
How many grams of boric acid should be used in this prescription to make the solution isotonic?
	Sodium chloride equivalent of Phenacaine = 0.17
	Sodium chloride equivalent of of Chlorbutanol = 0.18
	Sodium chloride equivalent of boric acid = 0.52
	
	1. Calculate the amount of phenacaine and chlorbutanol in the prescription: Phenacaine = 1% x 60mL = 0.6 g
	                  Chlorbutanol = 0.5% x 60 mL = 0.3g
	
	a. Find amount of NaCl represented by the ingredients in 60 mL
	           Phenacaine 0.17 x 0.6 = 0.102

> Chlorbutanol 0.18 x 0.3   = *0.054*
> Equivalence of NaCl represented   = 0.156 g
> b. How many g NaCl would have been required in 60 mL to make the solution isotonic: 0.9 % x 60 mL = 0.540 g
> c. How many grams of NaCl should be added:
> 0.540-0.156   = 0.384 g
> d. Since the prescription calls for boric acid, how much boric acid is required in place of NaCl:
> $\frac{0.384g}{0.52}$ = 0.738 g of boric acid. Answer.

13.4.1 Calculation of sodium chloride equivalents using Freezing point data.

Sodium Chloride equivalent can also be found by the following formula:

Sodium chloride equivalent of a substance = $\frac{FPD \text{ of substance in a solution of a given concentration}}{FPD \text{ of sodium chloride of the same concentration}}$

Where FPD = Freezing point depression.

For example, 1% ascorbic acid solution depress the freezing point of water by 0.105°C

1% sodium chloride solution depress the freezing point of water by 0.576°C

(in other words freezing point of 1% ascorbic acid and that of 1% sodium chloride solutions are - 0.105°C and -0.576°C respectively)

Therefore sodium chloride equivalent of ascorbic acid = $\frac{0.105}{0.576}$ = 0.18

Note that FPD is not proportional to concentration. Thus the table of sodium chloride equivalents gives values of sodium chloride equivalents for several concentrations (0.5%, 1%,2% 3% and 5%), and their freezing point depressions.

In calculations requiring sodium chloride equivalents based on freezing point data, just use the nearest value to the concentration in question in the FPD table. Table 5 lists o choice of freezing points of solutions of our interest, but the complete table has almost 300 medicaments at various concentrations.

To find the concentration of sodium chloride required to render a solution of a given medicament isotonic with body fluids,

> Step 1: look up in the table the sodium chloride equivalent for the strength nearest to the strength of medicament in preparation. When looking for the freezing point depression in the table,

> Step 2: Multiply the value in step 1 by the strength of the medicament

Step 3: subtract the result of step2 from 0.9 per cent (this is the concentration of sodium chloride which is isotonic with plasma). This difference is the strength of sodium chloride necessary to adjust the solution of the medicament to be isotonic.

% sodium chloride for adjustment to isotonicity = 0.9-($\sum$% of medicaments x sodium chloride equivalent)

Step 4. When a substance other than sodium chloride is to be used to adjust for isotonicity, find the amount of sodium chloride required and divide it by sodium chloride equivalent of the chosen substance.

Q283. Find the percentage of sodium chloride required to render 0.5% potassium chloride isotonic. Sodium chloride equivalent of 1% KCl solution = 0.76.	*% of NaCl required = 0.9 – (0.5 x 0.76) = 0.52*
Q284. find the percentage of dextrose required to render 1% solution ephedrine chloride isotonic.(sodium chloride equivalent of dextrose = 0.18)	*0.9 – (1 x 0.3) = 0.6 (NaCl)* $\frac{0.6}{0.18} = 3.3\%\ Dextrose$
Q285. What percentage of sodium chloride should be used to make 30 mL of a solution containing 2% cocaine HCl (i = 0.17), 2% Eucatropine HCl (i = 0.22) and 0.33% chlorbutanol (i = 0.18) isotonic with plasma?	% NaCl = 0.9-($\sum$% of medicaments x NaCl equivalent) = 0.9 – ((2% x 0.17)+(2% x 0.22)+(0.33 x 0.18) = 0.9 – (0.34 + 0.44 + 0.06) = 0.9 – 0.84 = 0.06% Answer. Thus in 30 mL we need 0.06% x30 = 0.018 g
Q286. Calculate the amount of boric acid (i= 0.52) required to make 30 mL of a solution containing 0.1g tertacaine HCL (i = 0.19) and 0.05 g of zinc sulphate (i =0.16) isotonic with lachrymal fluid.	Conc. of tetracaine HCl = $\frac{0.1g}{30mL}$ x100 = 0.33% Conc. of ZincSO$_4$ = $\frac{0.05g}{30mL}$ x100 = 0.17% % NaCl = 0.9-($\sum$% of medicaments x NaCl equivalent) = 0.9- ((0.33 x 0.19)+(0.17 x 0.16) = 0.9 – (0.06 + 0.03) = 0.9 -0.09 = 0.81% NaCl 0.81% means 0.81 g in 100 mL. How much should

	be in 30 mL: $\frac{0.81}{100} \times 30 = 0.243$ g of NaCl
	But we are required to use boric acid.
	Amount of boric acid required
	$= \frac{amount\ of\ NaCl}{NaCl\ equivalent\ of\ boric\ acid} = \frac{0.243}{0.52}$
	$= 0.467g$ Boric acid. Answer

13.5 TO FIND AMOUNT FOR ISOTONICITY USING FREEZING POINT DATA

Blood plasma and other body fluids such as lachrymal fluid, freeze at – 0.52° C. Any other solution that freezes at this temperature is isotonic with body fluids. Hypotonic fluids freeze at higher temperature. E.g. 1% procaine hydrochloride solution freezes at – 0.122° C. To render this solution isotonic, another substance (**the adjusting substance**) should be added so as to make the solution freeze at – 0.52° C. The adjusting substance should be able to lower the freezing point by 0.52-0.122 = 0.398.

Generally the proportion of the adjusting substance required to render the solution isotonic

$$- 0.52° C - \text{Freezing Point(FP) of the adjusting substance.}$$

A table is available that gives the Freezing point depressions (FPD) of 1% solutions of commonly used medicinal injections. Provided the solutions are fairly dilute, FPD of solutions are taken to be proportional to the concentrations (although this is not strictly true). Thus for a 0.5% and 1.5% or 2%, the FPD of 1% solution is halved, multiplied by 1.5 or multiplied by 2 respectively.

E.g. Freezing point of 1% adrenalin tartrate = - 0.098°C.
    Freezing point of 0.5% adrenaline tatrate = -0.049°C
        1.5% adrenaline tartrate = -0.147°C
        2% adrenaline tartrate = -0.196°C

Q287. 1% Procaine HCl solution freezes at -0.122°C. Calculate the amount of sodium chloride required to render 0.1 % procaine HCl isotonic with blood plasma. (1% sodium chloride freezes at 0.576°C)	If the freezing point (FP) of 1% procaine HCl is-0.122°C, The amount of NaCl required is the one capable of depressing the freezing point to -0.52°C that is a further 0.52-0.122= 0.398 1% NaCl solution depress the freezing point by 0.576°C What percent would depress the freezing point by 0.398? $\frac{1\%}{x\%} = \frac{0.576}{0.398}$ $X = \frac{0.398\ \times\ 1}{0.576}$ = 0.69% Answer.

Percentage w/v of adjusting substance needed $= \dfrac{0.52-a}{b}$

Where **a** = freezing point depression of the solution which should be adjusted for isotonicity

b = Freezing point depression of 1% w/v solution of the adjusting substance

** Note that solutes exert their effects independently and therefore the freezing point depressions (FDP) are summable. Each solute exerts its effect on freezing point independent of others present. Hence if two or more substances are present, **a** is the sum of their depressions.

Q288. The freezing point of 1% solution procaine HCl is -0.122°C. What concentration of procaine HCl is isotonic with blood plasma?	**Method 1:** *1% freezes at -0.122°C. What concentration would freeze at -0.52°C?* $\dfrac{1\%}{x\%} = \dfrac{0.122}{0.52}$ $X = \dfrac{0.52 \times 1}{0.122}$ X= 4.26% Answer **Method 2:** $\dfrac{0.52-a}{b} = \dfrac{0.52-0.00}{0.122} = 4.26\%$
Q289. How much sodium chloride should be added to 1.5% procaine hydrochloride iso-osmotic with blood plasma? (freezing point of 1% procaine HCl is -0.122°C	%NaCl required $= \dfrac{0.52-a}{b}$ a = freezing point of 1.5% procaine HCl FP of 1% procaine HCl x 1.5 = 0.122°C x 1.5 b= Freezing point of 1% NaCl solution = 0.576°C %NaCl required $= \dfrac{0.52-(0.122 \times 1.5)}{0.576} = 0.585\%$ w/v Answer
Q290. How many g of sodium chloride are required in 100 mL of 0.3% solution of zinc sulphate so that when this solution is diluted with an equal quantity of water becomes isotonic with body fluids? Freezing point of 1% ZnSO₄= -0.086°C Freezing point of 1% NaCl = -0.576°C	The quantity 100 mL must be made with double isotonic concentration, so that when it is diluted with an equal quantity of water it becomes a normal isotonic solution. **Method 1:** base the calculation on twice the freezing point depression: The formula $\dfrac{0.52-a}{b}$ becomes $\dfrac{(2 \times 0.52)-a}{b}$ %NaCl required = $\dfrac{(2 \times 0.52)-(0.3 \times 0.086)}{0.576}$ = 1.76 g in 100 mL Answer. **Method 2:** Base the calculation on the diluted solution 200 mL. Calculate the amount of sodium chloride required in 200 mL of the diluted solution. The concentration of zinc sulphate in the final solution 200 mL will be halved, instead of 0.3% it will be 0.15% $\dfrac{0.52-a}{b} = \dfrac{0.52-(0.15 \times 0.086)}{0.576} = 0.88\%$ 0.88% means 0.88 g in 100 mL therefore in 200 mL there are 1.76 g Answer

	Method 3:: Work out normally, ignoring the dilution. After 100 mL are made, plan to dilute with 0.9% sodium chloride solution with is isotonic:
	$\frac{0.52-a}{b} = \frac{0.52-(0.3 \times 0.086)}{0.576} = 0.86\%$
	In 100 mL 0.86 g is required. In another 100 mL, 0.9 g of sodium chloride is required, making a total of 0.88+0.9=1.76 g
	** The methods can be applied for other concentrations such as triple or quadruple dilutions prescribed.

13.6 CALCULATION FOR ISOTONICITY BASED ON MOLAR CONCENTRATION.

At normal temperature and pressure, a solution containing 1 g molecule of a non-ionizing solute in 22.4 liters has osmotic pressure of 1 atmosphere. Therefore in 1 liter, the solution containing 1 g molecular weight exerts osmotic pressure 22.4 atmospheres. In other words, 1 mole / Liter of a solutions exerts osmotic pressure of 22.4 atmospheres.

Osmotic pressure of blood plasma and lachrymal fluid is 6.7 atmospheres per liter. If one mole exerts 22.4 atmospheres per liter, we can calculate the molarity of plasma. It is actually $\frac{22.4}{6.7}$ = 0.3M.

Consequently any 0.3 M solution of a non-ionizing solute is isotonic.

General Formula: Concentration needed for isotonicity, $w = \frac{0.3M}{N}$

Where **M** is the molecular weight

And **N** is the number of ions per mole for ionizing substances.

Q291. 1 mole of dextrose is 180 g /L. Find the concentration of dextrose that is isotonic with blood plasma	$W = \frac{0.3M}{N}$ Dextrose does not ionize. Isotonic solution of dextrose therefore contains $\frac{0.3 \times 180}{1} = 54\ g/l\ or\ 5\%.$
Q292. Boric acid has a molecular weight of 62. Calculate the concentration of boric acid that is isotonic with blood plasma.	$W = \frac{0.3M}{N}$ $= \frac{(0.3 \times 62)}{1} = 8.6\ g/l\ or\ 1.86\%.$

Q293. Sodium chloride (Molecular weight W = 58.5) dissociates into 2 ions. Therefore N = 2. Calculate the concentration of sodium chloride which is isotonic with blood plasma	$W = \frac{0.3M}{N} = \frac{0.3 \times 58.5}{2} = 8.8\ g/L$ = approx. 0.9%
Q294. How much dextrose (M wt = 180) is required to make a 0.12 % solution of sodium chloride (Mol Wt 58.5) isotonic?	For sodium chloride, M = 58.5, It dissociates into 2 ions, therefore N = 2 Concentration of NaCl, W = 0.12%, = 1.2 g/L. Molarity of 1.2g/L NaCl = $\frac{1.2}{(58.5)} \times 2 = 0.041\ M$ But for isotonic solution, molarity should be 0.3M Therefore we still need 0.3-0.041 = 0.259 M of dextrose $\qquad = 0.259 \times 180\ g$ $\qquad = 46.62\ g/L$ or 4.66% w/v

Q295.
 ℞:
 Dextrose   2%
 Potassium Chloride   0.5%
 Sodium Chloride   q.s.
 Water Ad   500 mL
 	
 How many grams of sodium chloride are required to make the above solution isotonic?
	Step 1: Find the number of moles of dextrose and KCl
	
	 2% of dextrose means 2 g in 100 mL, To get the number of moles find the concentration in 1000 mL
	
	 Therefore 2 x 10 in 1000mL = 10 g = $\frac{20}{180} M = 0.11M$
	
	 0.5% of potassium Chloride means 0.5 g in 100 mL
	 KCl dissociates into 2 ions
	 Therefore 0.5 x 5 in 1000 mL = 5g = $\frac{5}{74.5} \times 2M$
	 = 0.1342M
	 Total number of moles present
	 = 0.11 + 0.1342 = 0.2442M
	
	 Step 2: Number of moles still required 0.3-0.2442 = 0.0558
	 Step 3: find required NaCl concentration.
	      NaCl dissociates into 2 ions.
	
	 = $\frac{0.0558 \times 58.5}{2} = 1.632$
	               or 0.16% w/v Answer.
	
	 Amount of sodium chloride required in 500 mL
	 = 0.16 x 5 = 0.8g

Q296. Calculate the percentage of sodium chloride necessary to render an injection containing 2 % per cent of methoxamine hydrochloride isotonic with blood plasma. 1% solution of methoxamine	**Method 1: Use freezing point data:** $\frac{0.52-a}{b} = \frac{0.52-(0.15 \times 2)}{0.576} = \frac{0.22}{0.576} = \mathbf{0.38\%}$ **Method 2: Use molecular concentration data:** Methoxamine HCL yields 2 ions on dissociation, Mol wt =247.7 2 % means 20 g in 1000 mL

HCl freezes at -0.15°C 1% NaCl solution freezes at -0.576°C Molecular weight of methoxamine hydrochloride = 247.7 Molecular weight of sodium chloride = 58.5	Number of moles of methoxamine present $= \frac{20}{247.2} \times 2$ $= 0.1615$ Required number of moles of adjusting substance $= 0.3 - 0.1615 = 0.1385$ Amount of sodium chloride required = 0.1385 moles. But NaCl is an electrolyte dissociating into 2 ions. Therefore the number of grams of NaCl required $= \frac{0.1385 \times 58.5}{2}$ $= 4\ g\ per\ liter\ or\ 0.40\%$ **Method 3:** Calculate the sodium chloride equivalent of methoxamine HCl **Sodium chloride equivalent of a substance =** $$\frac{FPD\ of\ substance\ in\ a\ solution\ of\ a\ given\ concentration}{FPD\ of\ sodium\ chloride\ of\ the\ same\ concentration}$$ $\frac{0.15}{0.576} = 0.26$ % of NaCl for adjustment = 0.9 – (2% x 0.26) = 0.9 – 0.52 = 0.38%

13.7 CALCULATION FOR ISOTONICITY BASED ON MILLIEQUIVALENTS

A liter of blood plasma on average contains 155 Milliequivalent of anions (mainly Na^+, K^+, Ca^{++} and Mg^{++}) and 155 milliequivalents of cations (mainly HCO^- Cl^- HPO_4^{2-}, SO_4^{2-}, proteins and organic acids). The ionic concentration of plasma is therefore 155 + 155 = 310 mEq/L.

Any solution containing solutes totaling 310 Milliequivalent / liter is isotonic with blood plasma. This provides another method of calculating amount of substances required to make any solution isotonic with blood plasma.

In order to find the amount of a substance to be added to a solution to adjust for isotonicity the general formula applies:

$b = 310 - a$

Where a = Number of mEq/L of a medicament in solution
And b = Number of mEq/L required of adjusting substance required

Q297. Calculate the amount of sodium chloride required to adjust a solution containing 40 mEq of potassium chloride.	$b = 310 - a$ $a = 80$ (40 mEq of KCl contain 40 mEq of K and 40 mEq of Cl, total = 80)

	$b = 310 - 80 = 230$
	
	NaCl is a two-ion electrolyte. Therefore if we need 230 mEq, they can be supplied by 115 mEq of NaCl (which supplies 115 mEq Na^+ and 115 mEq of Cl^-
	
	Equivalent weight of sodium chloride is 58.5.
	
	Therefore the amount of sodium chloride required
	$= 115 \times 58.5 = 6.73 \ g/L$
	
	The formula for the solution is:
	
	    Potassium chloride 74.5×40 = 2.98 g
	    Sodium chloride 58.5×115 = 6.73 g
	    Water Ad 1000 mL

Q298. Calculate the amount of sodium chloride required to make the following solution isotonic with blood plasma:
 	
Potassium chloride 0.3 g
Calcium chloride 0.29 g
Sodium chloride q.s
Water for injection, to 1000mL
	Step 1: Calculate the number of mEq of each component
	    Potassium chloride $\frac{300mg}{74.5} = 4 \ mEq$
	    KCl dissociates into 2 ions. Thus there are 8 mEq
	    Calcium chloride $\frac{290mg}{73.5} = 4 \ mEq$
	    $CaCl_2$ dissociates into approx. 2 ions supplying 8 mEq
	In total these provide 16 mEq.
	Step 2 Calculate the amount of sodium chloride required to adjust to isotonicity:
	    $b = 310 - a$
	Therefore Sodium chloride must be able to supply
	    $310 - 16 = 294 \ mEq$
	But NaCl dissociates into 2 ions.
	Thus, 294 mEq will be furnished by $294 \div 2 = 147 \ mEq$
	Equivalent weight of NaCl = 58.5
	Amount of NaCl required for isotonicity
	    $= 147 \times 58.5mg = 8599.5mg$ or 8.6 g Answer.

CHAPTER 14
Thermometry

14.1 Introduction

Simply put, **thermometry** means "measurement of temperature". Temperature is a very important aspect in pharmacy. Rates of chemical reactions, Industrial processing activities, deterioration of medicines and expression of febrile conditions can be monitored using temperature. Obtaining a patient's body temperature is a routine part of data collection. It is a well-known fact that accurate measurement provides useful clues about the severity of the illness.

14.2 Scales of Temperature>

Temperature is measured using a thermometer. There are two scales of temperature measurements namely **Fahrenheit (°F)** and **Centigrade (°C)** scales. The International Unit of temperature measurement is Centigrade. Sometimes it is called Celsius (from its inventor Anders Celsius). But Fahrenheit scale is still in use in many countries including USA and UK. As you may likely get involved in working with any of the scales at one point or another, it is important to be conversant with both scales and be able to interconvert them when the need arises.

In Fahrenheit scale (invented by a German scientist Gabriel Fahrenheit in 1709) the freezing point of water is -32°F and the boiling point of water is 212°F, a difference of 180° (212-32=180).

In Centigrade scale (introduced by a Swedish astronomer Anders Celsius in 1742), the freezing point of water is 0°C and the boiling point of water is 100°C, a difference of 100° (100-0=100).

Another scale known as **Kelvin scale** is of more interest to physics (and in medicinal chemistry). In this scale, the temperature -273°C or -459.4°F is known as Absolute Zero, as at this temperature there is practically no molecular activity theoretically.

The proportion of {Centigrade:Fahrenheit} can thus be devised using the difference between Fahrenheit and centigrade scale (as far as freezing and boiling of water are concerned):

$$\frac{Centigrade}{Fahrenheit} = \frac{100}{180} = \frac{5}{9}$$

This means for every 5° change in Centigrade thermometer, there is a corresponding 9° change in Fahrenheit thermometer.

Facts to remember:

Water freezes at 0°C or 32°F.

Body temperature is typically 37°C or 98.6°F

Water boils at 100°C or 212°F.

At -40 both temperatures are equal i.e. -40°F = -40°C

Absolute zero on Kelvin Scale -273°C = -459.4°F

Thus -273°C = -459.4°F	
-40°F = -40°C	
0°C = 32°F	
100°C =212°F	

14.2.1 Converting Centigrade to Fahrenheit

Method 1:

Using the fact that on Kelvin Scale, $-273°C = -459.4°F$

The ratio $\dfrac{Centigrade}{Fahrenheit}$ is equal to $\dfrac{C+273}{F+459.4} = \dfrac{5}{9}$

$$9(C+273) = 5(F+459.4)$$

> Thus $C = \dfrac{5}{9}(F + 459.4) - 273$
>
> And $F = \dfrac{9}{5}(C + 273) - 459.4$

Method 2: Use the fact that $-40°F = -40°C$

Thus $\dfrac{Centigrade}{Fahrenheit}$ is equal to $\dfrac{C+40}{F+40} = \dfrac{5}{9}$

$$9(C+40) = 5(F+40)$$

> $$C = \dfrac{5}{9}(F + 40) - 40$$
>
> $$F = \dfrac{9}{5}(C + 40) - 40$$

Method 3: Standard Method

Use the fact that $-32°F = 0°C$

$\dfrac{Centigrade}{Fahrenheit}$ is equal to $\dfrac{C}{F-32} = \dfrac{5}{9}$

$$9C = 5(F-32)$$

> $$C = \dfrac{5}{9}(F - 32)$$
>
> $$F = 32 + \dfrac{9}{5}C$$

Method 4: (Easiest method)

It is a fact that whichever proportion, as long as the proportions are equal, multiplying the means and extremes simply gives the same equation:

Let us look at method 1 through 3:

Method 1: $\dfrac{C+273}{F+459.4} = \dfrac{5}{9}$ 9(C+273) =5(F+459.4) → 9C +2457 = 5F + 2297 ⟶ **9C=5F-160**

Method 2: $\dfrac{C+40}{F+40} = \dfrac{5}{9}$ 9(C+40) = 5(F+40) → 9C +360 = 5F -160 ⟶ **9C=5F-160**

Method 3: $\dfrac{C}{F-32} = \dfrac{5}{9}$ 9 C = 5(F-32) ⟶ ⟶ **9C=5F-160**

This is the easiest method. It is easy to remember, it is simple hence prevents errors that may arise due to careless interchange of 9/5 or 5/9 and it has no confusion of minus or plus signs that appear in other equations. What is important is understanding the principles involved in arriving at the equation.

Please note that when Centigrade degrees are converted to Fahrenheit, fractions are fifths and are customarily expressed as decimals. However, when Fahrenheit degrees are converted to Centigrade, fractions are ninths.

Q299. Convert 15°C to Fahrenheit	*9C=5F-160* *9x15 =5F -160* *135 + 160 = 5F* *5F= 295* *F = 59°*
Q300. Convert -25°C to Fahrenheit	*9C=5F-160* *9 x -25 = 5F -160* *-225 +160 = 5F* *5F = -65* *F = -13°*
Q301. Convert 32°F to centigrade	*9C=5F-160* *9C =(5x32)-160* *9C = 160 -160 =0* $C = \dfrac{9}{0} =$ *0°*
Q302. Convert 87°F to Centigrade scale	*9C=5F-160* *9C = (5x87)-160* *9C = 435 -160 = 275* $C = \dfrac{275}{9} =$ $30\dfrac{5}{9}°$

Chapter 15

CALCULATIONS INVOLVING INJECTABLES AND RECONSTITUTION OF POWDERED MEDICATIONS

15.1 Introduction

This chapter is deals with calculations associated with rates of flow of intravenous fluids and administration of insulin and heparin. It also deals with reconstitution of powdered medications as well as aspects of Milliequivalent and milliosmoles as related to injectable medications.

Intravenous fluids (IV drips) must be precisely regulated to ensure adequate hydration of patients. Usually administration equipment state the *Drop factor* (drops per mL) it delivers e.g. 10, 15, or 20 drops per mL. Microdropper (or minidroppers) sets deliver 60 drops/mL. Blood transfusion sets usually deliver 15 drops/mL.

15.2 Calculation of rate of flow of intravenous fluids

The rate of infusion of IV drips is calculated using the following formula:

R = Number of drops per Minute (Rate of flow) (gtt per min) =

$$\frac{\text{Number of mL to be infused} \times \text{drops per mL (or drop factor)}}{\text{number of hours for adm} \times \text{60 minutes per hour}}$$

GENERALLY, $\quad R = \frac{V \times D}{T}$

Where R = Rate of flow (gtt/min)
V = total volume to be infused (in mL)
D = drop factor (gtt/mL)
T = total time of infusion (in minutes)

Q303. Calculate the IV flow rate for 500 mL D5W to run for 8 hours at a drop factor of 60 gtt/mL	$R = \frac{V \times D}{T} R = \frac{500 \times 60}{8 \times 60} = \frac{30,000}{480}$ = 62.5 gtt/min. answer
Q304. One liter of an infusion bag contains 2.5 million units of ampicillin. How many units will have been infused after 6 hours with a flow rate of 1.2 ml minute	Total volume delivered after 6 hours = 1.2 ml /min 60 min x 6 hrs. = 432 ml There are 2,500,000units in 1000 mL. How units many are in 432 mL? $\frac{432}{1000} \times 2{,}500{,}000 = 1{,}080{,}000$ Units. Answer

Q305. 1 liter of Ringer's injection (IV fluid) was started at 10 pm. After 7 hours it was found that 800 mL still remained. The clinic is supposed to close 5 hour later. Calculate the flow rate (in drops/min and mL/min) that must be set to complete the administration in the remaining time if the IV set delivers 15 drops/mL	*Fluid remaining = 800 mL,* *Time remaining = 5 hours (or 300 minutes)* $R = \frac{V \times D}{T} = \frac{800 \text{ mL} \times 15}{5 \times 60} = 40 \text{ drops /min}$ *If 800 mL are infused in 300 min, calculate the number of mL per minute using proportions:* $\frac{800mL}{XmL} = \frac{300min}{1min}$ $X = 2.67 \text{ mL/min Answer}$
Q306. ℞ 1000 mL D5W IV 24 hr. Using a microdrop set that delivers 60 drops /mL, calculate the flow rate (drops/min and mL/min) of the infusion	$R = \frac{V \times D}{T} = \frac{1000 \text{ mL} \times 60 gtt \text{ per mL}}{24 \text{ hr} \times 60 \text{ minutes}}$ *=42 gtt/min Answer.* *Also 1000 mL are infused over 24hr x 60 min = 1440 minutes. How many mL are infused per mL?:* $\frac{1000mL}{1mL} = \frac{1440minutes}{XmL}$ *X = 0.69 mL,* *The rate = 0.69mL/min Answer.* *From mL/min, you can also calculate gtt/min as follows:* *60 drops are in 1 mL, how many drops are in 0.69mL?. Then by proportion:* $\frac{60 \text{ drops}}{X \text{ drops}} = \frac{1mL}{0.69mL}$ *X = 42 gtt/min*
Q307. An IV set delivers 10 drops per mL. If 1 Liter of D5W solution is administered for 8 hrs., calculate the number of drops per minute.	$R = \frac{V \times D}{T} = \frac{1000mL \times 10gtt \text{ per mL}}{8hrs \times 60 \text{ minutes}} = 20.8 \frac{gtt}{min}$ *=Approx. 21 drops per minute. Answer.* *Also 1000 mL are infused over 480 minutes (=8 hrs.). How many Ml are infused in 1 minute?:* $\frac{1000}{X} = \frac{480}{1}$ *X = 2.08 mL/min* *If 10 drops = 1 mL, How many drops are in 2.08 mL?:* $\frac{10 \text{ drops}}{X \text{ drops}} = \frac{1 mL}{2.08 mL}$ *X = 21 drops*

15.3 Calculation of dosage of Insulin

Insulin is a hormone produced by pancreas and responsible for carbohydrate, protein and fat metabolism. Absence or lack of this essential hormone leads to development of Diabetes disease. Insulin therefore is a drug that is used in the treatment of type 1 diabetes and occasionally in type 2 diabetes when the need arises.

Insulin is classified either according to the duration of action (i.e. rapid acting; intermediate acting or Long acting) or according to its source (e.g. human insulin, porcine insulin and beef insulin). The strength or potency of insulin and hence its dose is expressed in terms of units of activity per mL.

There are four types of Insulin syringes namely:
1. Standard U-100 syringe (marked every 2 units up to 100 units)
2. 1-mL 100 insulin syringe (marked for every 1 unit up to 100 units)
3. The 50-unit Lo-Dose U-100 insulin syringe (easier to read and used for low dose of insulin)
4. The 30-unit LO-Dose Insulin syringe (reads up to 30 units and is the most accurate for measurement of small amounts of insulin especially in children.

Q308. ℞/: U-40 Isophane Insulin Suspension 10 Units U-100 Protamine Zinc Insulin 18 units What volume (in mL) of each type is required to provide the desired dose?	U-40 insulin contains 40 units/mL. How many mL contain 10 units? $\frac{40\ units}{10\ units} = \frac{1 mL}{X mL}$ $X = 0.25\ mL$ U-100 Insulin contains 100 units/mL. How many mL contain 18 units? $\frac{100\ units}{18\ units} = \frac{1\ mL}{X\ mL}$ $X = 0.18\ mL$ Therefore we need 0.25 mL of U-40 and 0.18mL of U-100 Insulin. Answer
Q309. How many mL of U-100 Insulin (Regular) should be used to obtain 60 units?	U-100 mL contains 100 units/mL. How many mL contain 60 units? $\frac{100}{60} = \frac{1}{X}$ $X = 0.6 mL$ Answer

15.4 Calculation of Heparin Dosage

Heparin, an anticoagulant that prevents formation of clots of blood, just like insulin, is measured in *units of activity*. The normal heparinising dosage for adults is 20,000 to 40,000 units per day (24 hrs.), administered as IV *units per hour* or as per physician request, as mL per hour.

Q310. A patient undergoing hip surgery was prescribed heparin at a dose of 120 units/kg body weight. How many mL of heparin (5000 units/mL) should be administered to a 100 kg person?	Total Units required = 120 Units/kg x 100kg = 12000 Units. Each mL contains 500 units. How many mL contain 12000 units? $\frac{5000\ units}{12000\ units} = \frac{1\ mL}{x\ mL}$ $X = 2.4\ mL$
Q311. Calculate the number of units/mL if a 4 mL	Total number of units = 4 mL x 10,000 units

vial of heparin containing 10,000 units/mL is injected in 1 liter bottle of NS	$= 40{,}000$ units 1000 mL contain 40,000 units 1 mL contains ? units $\dfrac{1{,}000}{1\,mL} = \dfrac{40{,}000\ units}{X\ Units} \quad X = 40\ units$

15.5 Calculation involving Reconstitution of Dry Powders

Penicillins (e.g. Ampicillin, amoxicillin and cloxacillin) and some other antibiotics (such as erythromycin, cefalexin, cefuroxim and chloramphenicol) are affected by water in solution. Therefore they are prepared as dry powders to be reconstituted just prior to use. After reconstitution, it is recommended that they are used within a week to avoid deterioration. If the medications are intended for use as injections, a sterile diluent such as water for injection or normal saline is admixed in a specified volume as stated on the label to achieve a specified concentration.

Q312. How many mL of water for injection should be added to a vial containing 200,000 units of Penicillin G potassium in order to prepare a solution having a concentration of 25,000 units/mL?	If the final solution has 25,000 units/mL, how many mL should be added to 200,000 units to achieve the same concentration?: $\dfrac{25{,}000\,Units}{200000\,Units} = \dfrac{1mL}{XmL} \quad X = 8mL$
Q313. ℞: Pen G 300,000 IU in 500 mL D5W How many mL of Pen G reconstituted solution must be added to the 500 mL D5W infusion? The label on the drip reads : " Penicillin G Potassium 1,000,000 Units. Directions: Add Diluent 4.6 mL to achieve a concentration of solution 200.000 units/ mL"	In the final solution, there are 200,000 units per mL. How many mL contain 300,000 units? $\dfrac{200000\ units}{300000\ units} = \dfrac{1\ mL}{X\ mL} \quad X = 1.5\ mL$
Q314. Rocephin ® injection (Ceftriaxone) is available as 250 mg, 500 mg and 1 g vials, to be reconstituted using 2 mL, 2mL and 2,5 mL respectively. After reconstitution, the final volume is 2 mL, 2.2 mL and 3 mL respectively. Calculate the number of mL required for each package if the dose of ceftraxone is 7 mg/kg for a 56-kg patient .	The amount of drug required for a 56 kg patient Is $7 \times 56 = 392$ mg. From a 250 mg vial (which has 2 mL after reconstitution,.: 2 mL = 250 mg ? mL = 392 mg $\dfrac{2}{x} = \dfrac{250}{392} \quad X = 3.1\ mL$ From a 500 mg vial, which has 2.2 mL after reconstitution $\dfrac{2.2}{X} = \dfrac{500}{392} \quad X = 1.7\ mL$

	From a 1g vial, which has 3 mL, $\frac{3}{X} = \frac{1000}{392}$ $x = 1.2\ mL$	
Q315. A package contains 5 g penicillin V powder. When reconstituted, it makes 200 mL. How many mg of the medicine is in each 5 ml of the dose?	$\frac{5g}{X} = \frac{200mL}{5mL}$	$X = 0.125\ g = 125\ mg$

15.6 Milliequivalents and Milliosmoles in injectable solutions

Calculations involving Milliequivalent, Millimole and milliosmoles were covered in detail in chapters 12 through 13. This section highlights calculations relevant to injections. To recapitulate,

$$1\ mEq = \frac{Molecular\ wt}{valence \times number\ of\ particles}$$

Number of Milliequivalent $= \dfrac{wt\ of\ a\ substance\ (in\ mg)}{milli\ equivalent\ wt\ (expressed\ in\ mg)}$

15.6.1 Calculation involving Milliequivalent in injectables.

Q316. How much calcium chloride ($CaCl_2.2H_2O$) (Mol Wt = 147) is required to provide 2,5 mEq Ca^{2+}	$1\ mEq = \frac{147}{2} = 73.5\ mg.$ $2.5\ mEq = 73.5 \times 2.5 = 183.75\ mg$
Q317. A 55kg patient was prescribed Potassium chloride 0.25 mEq per kg body weight, to be added to a 500 ml drip of dextrose. How many mL of 50 mEq/10 mL sterile Potassium chloride should be used to provide the required potassium chloride?	Quantity of KCl required = 0.25 mEq × 55kg = 13.75 mEq The solution contains 50 mEq per 10 mL. Calculate how many mL contain 13.75 mEq: $\frac{50}{13.75} = \frac{10}{X}$ $X = 2.75\ mL$ Answer

Q318.
KH_2PO_4 0.75 g (Mol wt = 136)
             (Eq wt = 136 g)
K_2HPO_4 3.5 g   (Mol wt =174)
             (Eq wt = 87 g)
Water for inj.   ad   10 mL
 	
5 mL of the above solution was added to 1000 mL D5W. How many mEq of potassium phosphate were in the final solution?
	Number of mEq of $KH_2PO_4 = \frac{wt(mg)}{Eq\ wt(mg)} = \frac{750mg}{136mg}$
	$= 5.51\ mEq$
	
	Number of mEq of $K_2HPO_4 = \frac{3500mg}{87mg} = 40.23\ mEq$
	In 10 mL there are 5.51 + 40.23 = 45.74 mEq of potassium phosphate.
	In 5 mL of the solution (which were added to 1000 mLD5W) there are $45.74 \times \frac{5}{10} = 22.87\ mEq$ Ans.

15.6.2 Calculations involving milliosmoles

Addition of electrolytes in the body affects the osmotic pressure and hence the movement of fluids from and to the cells. Electrolytes establish osmotic pressure responsible for the movement of fluid between intercellular and extracellular spaces. The osmotic pressure is proportional to the number of particles (the molecules or ions of electrolytes) and is expressed in units of **milliosmoles (mOsm) per liter.** For non-electrolytes,

$$\text{Osmol/L} = \frac{g.\,of\,solute\,per\,liter}{Gram\,mol\,wt\,of\,solute} \times 1000$$

Electrolytes dissociate into individual ions according to the dissociation constant. The Osmolar concentration of electrolytes is calculated using the following formula:

$$\text{MOsmol/L} = \frac{(g\,of\,solute\,per\,liter) \times (Number\,of\,ions\,formed)}{gram\,Mol\,wt\,of\,solute} \times 1000$$

The milliosmolar value of separate ions of an electrolyte =

$$\frac{Concentration\,of\,the\,ion\,(mg\,per\,L)}{atomic\,wt\,of\,the\,ion}$$

The milliosmolar value of the whole electrolyte equals to the sum of the milliosmolar values of all the ions in the solution. All substances in a solution contribute independently to the overall osmotic pressure of the solution.

Q319. Calculate the number of mOsmol represented in 1 liter of normal saline (0,9% Sodium chloride). Mol wt of NaCl = 58.5	1000 mL of 0.9% NaCl contain 9 g of NaCl. There are 2-ions, Na^+ and Cl^- mOsmol/L = $\frac{(g\,of\,solute\,per\,liter) \times (Number\,of\,ions\,formed)}{gram\,Mol\,wt\,of\,solute} \times 1000$ $= \frac{9 \times 2}{58.5} \times 1000 = 308\,Osmol/L$ Ans.
Q320. Calculate the osmolarity of a solution containing 0.45% NaCl and 5% dextrose. (Mol wt NaCl = 58.5, Mol wt Dextrose =180)	Osmolarity = mOsmol/L 0.45 % NaCl means 4.5 g per L. Number of mOsmol/L NaCl $= \frac{4.5 \times 2}{58.5} \times 1000 = 153.8$ 5% dextrose means 50 g per liter. Dextrose does not dissociate. Number of mOsmol $= \frac{50 \times 1}{180} \times 1000 = 277.8$ Total mOsmol = 153.8 + 277.8 = 431.6 mOsmol/L

CHAPTER 16

CALCULATIONS INVOLVING INTRAVENOUS NUTRITIONAL SUPPLIMENTATION

16.1 Introduction

Supplementation of nutrients is inevitable in patients with serious nutritional deficiencies and patients unable to eat due to diseases, extensive burns, complications and surgery. Patients who are unable to take food orally need Total parenteral nutrition (TPN), defined as provision of nutrients intravenously in sufficient amounts to maintain or achieve anabolism.

Assessment of the nutritional status can be done either subjectively (changes in weight, body functions, emaciating symptoms, history and disease metabolic demands) or by Prognostic Nutrition Index (PNI), which uses markers such as levels of serum albumin, and transferring; body fats, lean body mass and skinfold thickness.

Nutritional supplementation takes into account amount of nitrogen and calories that a given substance may provide, the protein-calorie percentage of a substance and use of parenteral hyperalimentation. A knowledge of Resting Energy Expenditure (REE) is also important to assess the amount of energy that should be provided by the food in total parenteral nutrition.

16.2 Calculation of calories

A calorie is a unit of energy (or heat), defined as energy needed to increase the temperature of 1 gram of water by 1°C at atmospheric pressure. In Nutrition, the unit commonly used is kilocalorie (kCal). One kCal =1000 calories, which is the energy required to raise the temperature of 1 kg of water by 1°C at atmospheric pressure. The SI unit for energy is the Joule. 1 kCal =4.184 kJ

Typically, the caloric density (= kCal/gram) of common nutritional substances are:

Glucose, anhydrous ($C_6H_{12}O$)	3.85 kCal/g
Glucose, monohydrate ($C_6H_{12}O_6 \cdot H_2O$)	3.40 kCal/g
Proteins	4.10 kCal/g
Fat Emulsions	9.0 kCal/g
Alcohol	7.0 kCal/g

Components of parenteral nutrition contribute their caloric value independent of each other and the total calories is the sum of calories contributed by individual components.

To calculate the number of calories in a given product, we need to calculate the number of grams of the substance in the package and multiply it by its caloric density.

Q321. How many Calories are in 2 liters of D5W?	Step 1: Find the amount of dextrose in 2 L D5W: Grams of dextrose = Volume (mL) x %

	dextrose $= 2000\ mL \times \frac{5}{100} = 100\ g$ Step 2: Multiply the wt by its caloric density: $100 \times 3.4 = 340\ kCal$
Q322. An IV solution for dietary supplement contains 20% carbohydrate, 10% protein and 6% fats. How many calories are in 3 liters of the solution?	Step 1: Calculate the quantity of each substrate in 3L (or 3000 mL) a) 20% glucose in $3\ L = 3000 \times \frac{20}{100} = 600\ g\ glucose$ b) 10% proteins $= 3000 \times \frac{10}{100} = 300\ g$ proteins c) 6% fats $= 3000 \times \frac{6}{100} = 180\ g\ fats$ Step 2 multiply the quantity and its respective caloric density: Glucose: 600 g x 3.4 kcal/g=2040 kcal Proteins: 300 g x 4.1 kcal/g = 1230 kcal Fats: 180 g x 9kcal/g = 1620 kcal Step 3: sum up all the calories: 2040 + 1230 + 1620 = 4890 kcal. Answer.

16.3 Nitrogen, Calorie/Nitrogen Ratio, and Protein-Calorie percentage of TPN

The body requires proteins in order to synthesize tissues (anabolism). Proteins are made by our body by utilizing nitrogen. Nitrogen therefore is a very important component of diet and it must be provided in adequate amount. The lack of nitrogen (negative nitrogen balance) leads to emaciation, body wasting, failure to thrive (especially in children) and delay or failure to recover from diseases.

An adult person requires 0.8-1.5 g of protein per kg body weight everyday (56-105 g/day for 70kg person). 6.25 g of proteins or amino acids contain 1 g of nitrogen. In other words, nitrogen is 16% in proteins ($16\% = \frac{1}{6.25} \times 100$).

16.3.1 Nitrogen

Q323. How much nitrogen is required for a 70-kg person?	Amount of protein required = 0.8 -1.5 g/kg A 70 kg person requires (0.8 -1.5) x 70 $= 56g - 105\ g$, Nitrogen is 16% in proteins Thus amount of Nitrogen required $= 56 \times \frac{16}{100}$ to $105 \times \frac{16}{10}$ $= 9\ g\ to\ 17\ g$ answer.

Grams of nitrogen available from protein source = $Grams\ of\ protein \times \frac{16}{100}$

$$OR = \frac{grams\ of\ protein}{0.65}$$

Q324. How much nitrogen is in 1 L of 10% amino acid solution	Amount of amino acid = $1000 \text{ mL} \times \frac{10}{100}$ $= 100 \text{ g}$ $$\text{grams of nitrogen} = \frac{100}{6.25} = 16 \text{ g}$$

16.3.2 Calorie/Nitrogen Ratio

In order to understand this ratio consider One liter of a TPN solution made by combining 500 mL of 50% dextrose and 500 mL of 9% amino acid solution:

Amount of dextrose = $500 \times \frac{50}{100} = 250 \text{ g}$. It provides non-protein energy, equivalent to $250 g \times 3.4 \frac{kcal}{g} = 850 \text{ kcal}$

Grams of amino acid = $500 \times \frac{9}{100} = 45 \text{ g}$. Grams of nitrogen = $\frac{45}{6.25} = 7.2 \text{ g}$

The ratio of non-nitrogen protein to grams of nitrogen = $\frac{850 \, kcal}{7.2 \, g} = 118:1$

The calorie :Nitrogen ratio (as determined by dividing the total non-nitrogen calories to grams of nitrogen provided) promotes optimum nitrogen utilization for the synthesis of proteins. The optimal ratio is 100-200 non-nitrogen calories per gram of nitrogen. In unstressed patients the best ratio is 135-175. In severely stressed patients, it is lower.

Q325. Calculate the total calories available in 1000 mL of a solution containing 12.5% dextrose and 5% amino acids. What is the calorie/nitrogen ratio of this solution?	

16.3.3. Protein-calorie percentage.

Protein-calorie percentage = $\frac{\text{total number of calories from protein source}}{\text{total number of calories from all sources}} \times 100$

Q326. 1000 mL of a TPN solution contains 25% dextrose and 4.25 % proteins. Calculate the protein-calorie percentage of this solution.	Amount of calories from dextrose: $= 1000 \text{ mL} \times \frac{25}{100} \times 3.4 \text{ kcal per g} = 850 \text{ Kcal}$: Amount of calories from protein: $= 1000 \times \frac{4.25}{100} \times 4.1 \text{ kcal per g} = 174.25 \text{ kcal}$ Total calories = 850 +174.25= 1024.25 kcal. The protein calorie percentage = $\frac{174.25}{1024.25} \times 100$ = 17%

Chapter 16

Worked Examples.

Q327. How many grams of Dextrose is present in a 500mL D5W solution ?	500 mL of D5W (dextrose 5%) solution contains 500 x 5/100 = 25 gram of dextrose.
Q328. How many grams of drug is required to dispense 1 pint of 1 in 25 solution?	1 in 25 solution is interpreted as 1 gm of drug in 25mL solution, therefore we can say 1 pint (480mL) solution of drug will contain = 480/25 = 19.20 grams of drug.
Q329. How much lignocaine is present in 30 mL solution of a 1 :1000, solution of lignocaine ?	1 : 1000 means 1 gm of lignocaine in 1000mL of solution, therefore 30mL solution of lignocaine will present in = 30/1000 = 0.03 gram (30mg) lignocaine.
Q330. How much atropine is required to dispense 1 quart of 1 in 100 solution ?	1 in 100 contains 1 gram of drug in 100mL of solution. We want to prepare 1 quart (960mL), therefore 960/100 = 9.6 gram of drug.
Q331. How many mL of 75% alcohol should mix with 1000mL of 10% alcohol solution to prepare 500mL of 30% alcohol ?	Use alligation method. 75 20 (75%) 30 10 45 (10%) Total parts 65 (30%) We want to prepare 500mL 30% alcohol solution, therefore one can say To prepare 65 (30%) 20 (75%) parts To prepare 500 (30%) ? 500 x 20/65 = 153.84mL 75% solution is required.
Q332. How many milligrams are equal to 1/200 grain of nitroglycerine ?	1 grain is equal to 65 mg. Therefore 1/200 gr is equal to = 1/200 x 65 = 0.325mg
Q333. If 1 teaspoonful of Thioridazine intense solution (30mg/mL) is diluted up to 480mL mark with plain water, what would be the final strength of solution in mg/mL?	1 teaspoonful (5mL) will contain 150mg of Thioridazine (30mg/mL). This solution is diluted up to 480mL mark with plain water, therefore 150mg/480mL = 0.31mg/mL.
Q334. If 60 gram of 1% Hydrocortisone is mixed with 80 grams of 2.5% Hydrocortisone, what is the % w/w of hydrocortisone in final mixture?	The content of hydrocortisone is final mixture can be calculated by 60 gm of 1% Hydrocortisone = 0.6 gm 80 gm of 2.5% Hydrocortisone = 2.0 gm 140 gm of Hydrocortisone = 2.6 gm % of Hydrocortisone in final mixture 2.6 x100 140 = 1.85%

Q335. Find out the ratio of an ionize drug to unionize at pH = 7. The pKa value of drug is 5.	$pH = PKa + \log \frac{salt}{acid}$ $7 = 5 + \log \frac{salt}{acid}$ $2 = \log salt/acid$ $(salt/acid) = 10^{-2}$
Q336. An adult dose of drug is 500mg, what is the dose for a 2-year old child? (Young rule)	According to young formula $\frac{age\ in\ year}{(age + 12)} X\ Adult\ dose$ $= 2 \times \frac{2}{14} \times 500\ mg$ $= 71.42\ mg\ of\ drug.$
Q337. If an adult dose of drug is 750mg, what is the dose for child weighing 20 lbs.?	According to Clark formula $= \frac{weight\ (in\ lb.) \times adult\ dose}{150\ lbs.}$ $= 20 \times \frac{20}{150} \times 750\ mg = 100mg\ dose.$
Q338. If an adult dose of drug is 100mg, what would be dose for a child that has a body surface area 0.9 m²?	$\frac{Body\ surface\ area\ of\ child \times adult\ dose}{173\ m^2}$ $= \frac{0.9}{173} \times 100$ $= 0.52\ mg\ of\ dose.$
Q339. If therapeutic dose of drug is 10mg/kg/day, how many 250mg/100mL ready-infusions bags should be filled? Patient's weight is 156 lbs.	Patient weight in kg is 156lbs/2.2 = 70.9 kg. The therapeutic dose of the drug is 10mg/kg, so patient needs = 70.9 x 10 = 709 mg of the drug. Therefore the correct answer should be 3-bags.
Q340. How many mL of water should mix with 70% alcohol to prepare 750 mL of 20% alcohol?	Use alligation method. 70　　　　　　20 (70%) 　　　　20 0　　　　　　50 (0%) Total parts 70 (20%) To prepare 70 parts (20%) 50 parts (0%) So, to prepare 750 mL (20%)? = 750 x 50 / 70 = 535.71 mL of water should be mixed with 214.29 mL (750mL - 535.71mL) of 70% alcohol to prepare 750mL of 20% alcohol.
Q341. Aluminum (Al^{+3}) has a gram atomic weight of 27. What would be the Milliequivalent weight?	Milliequivalents of Al^{3+} ion = $Eq\ weight = \frac{atomic\ weight(g)}{valence}$ $= \frac{27g}{3}$ $= 9\ gm\ Equivalent\ weight$ $mEq = \frac{equivalent\ weight\ in\ mg}{1000}$

	$= \frac{9000}{1000} = 9$
Q342. How many mEq of Na+ presents in 250 mL of 0.9% of normal saline solution ? (MW = 58.5 gram/mole)	Milliequivalents of Na^+ $= \frac{molecular\ weight\ of\ NaCl\ (expressed\ as\ mg)}{valence}$ $= \frac{58.5}{1}$ $= 58.5\ mg$ Amount of NaCl in 250 mL of 0.9 % NaCl solution is = 250 x 0.009 = 2.25 gm, = 2250 mg Number of Milliequivalent of $Na^+ = \frac{2250}{58.5} = 38.36$
Q343. How many Milliequivalent of ferrous are present in 5 gr of ferrous sulfate? [MW = 152 gm/mole]	Eq wt of $FeSO_4 = \frac{gmolwt}{valence}$ $= \frac{152}{2} = 76\ gm$ mEq of $FeSO_4 = 76\ mg$ 1 gr = 0.065 g 5gr = 0.325 g = 325 mg Total $mEq = \frac{325\ mg}{76\ mg} = 4.27\ mEq$
Q344. An adult I.V. dose of Neupogen is 20mcg/kg/twice a week, how many milligrams will patient receive a week ? [patient weight = 150 lbs.]	Patient is weighing $\frac{150}{2.2}$ lbs = 68.18 kg A normal therapeutic dose in an adult patient is = 20 mcg x 68.18 kg = 1363 mcg per twice a week. = 681.81 mcg per a week. = 0.68 mg per a week.
Q345. If an I.V. admixture contains 1000mg of drug in 250 mL solution, how many drops per minute are required to infuse 50mg of drug per minute ? [I.V set delivers 20 drops/mL]	An I.V. admixture contains 1000mg of drug in 250mL of solution, therefore one can say $= \frac{1000mg}{250mL} = 4\ mg/mL$ I.V. set delivers 20 drops per mL, therefore to administer 50 mg dose of drug we require $= \frac{50 \times 20}{4}$ = 250 drops per minute.
Q346. Administration of 1.5 gram/kg/day of Amino acid normally achieves optimum fat metabolism and spares protein catabolism, what would be the dose of amino acids in grams/day for 155lbs patient ?	Patient weight is 155lb /2.2 = 70.45 kg A normal therapeutic dose is 1.5 gm x 70.45 kg = 105.68 gm of drug.
Q347. How many calories are provided by 500mL of D30W solution	500mL of D30W solution contains = 500 x 0.3 gm = 150 gm dextrose Each gm of dextrose provides =3.4 calories, therefore 150 gm dextrose will provide = 150 x 3.4 calories = 510 calories

Q348. What would be total calories provided by TPN mixture containing 1200mL D5W, 1000mL of 10% amino acids, 100mL of 5% alcohol and 300mL of 20% fat emulsion ?	1200mL of D5W provide = 1200 x 0.05 x 3.4 = 204 calories. 1000mL of 10% amino acid provide = 1000 x 0.1 x 4 = 400 calories. 100mL of 5% alcohol solution contains = 100 x 0.05 x 5.6 calories = 28 calories 1mL of 20% fat emulsion provides = 2 calories 300mL of 20% lipid solution will provide = 300 x 2 = 600 calories Total calories provide = 204+400+28+600
Q349. How many Milliequivalent of sodium are present in a 50mL 50% solution of sodium bicarbonate ? [MW = 84 gm/mole]	50mL of 50% sodium bicarbonate solution contains = 25 gm of sod bicarbonate. Eq weight = gm mole wt / valence = 84 gm / 1 = 84 g mEq = Eq wt / 1000 = 84 / 1000 = 0.084 g Total mEq of sod = 25 g / 0.084 g/Eq = 297.61 mEq
Q350. An adult recommended dose of drug is 5mg/kg/day, how many milligrams of drug is required every four hours? [patient weight =110 lbs.]	Patient weight in kg = 150 / 2.2 = 50 kg A normal recommended dose of drug per day is = 5 x 50 = 250mg per day. Patient is taking this dose in 6 divided doses, therefore every 4 hours dose of drug would be = 250mg/ 6 = 41.66mg every 4-hour.
Q351. If an I.V. order is for 250mL of D5W to be given every 6 hours, what would be the flow rate in drops/min? [I.V. set delivers 20 drops/mL]	We have 250mL of dextrose solution, which needs to be administered in 6 hours (360 minutes), therefore one can say In 360 minutes === 250mL solution In 1 minute ===== ? = 250 / 360 = 0.69 mL/min An I.V. set delivers 20 drops per mL, therefore 1 mL contains 20 drops 0.69 mL will need ? = 20 x 0.69mL = 13.8 drops/min = 14 drops/min
Q352. Find out the ratio of an ionize drug to unionize at pH = 7. The pKa value of drug is 5.	$pH = pKa + \log\frac{Salt}{Acid}$ $7 = 5 + \log\frac{Salt}{Acid}$ $2 = \log\frac{salt}{Acid}\frac{Salt}{Acid} = 10^{-2}$ Answer
Q353. Ammonium chloride (NH₄Cl – Mol wt 53.5) is to be used as a urinary acidifier with a dose of 150 Milliequivalent. How many tablets of 150 mg each should be administered	1 mEq = 53.5 mg 150 mEq = 53.5 x 150 mg The number of 150 mf tablets required = $\frac{53.3 \times 150}{150}$ = 53.5 tablets (We thus need 54 tablets)
Q354. How many milliliters of 17% benzalkonium chloride should be used to	1: 1500 = 1/1500x100 = 0.67% $C_1V_1 = C_2V_2$

prepare 500 mL of a solution containing 1:1500 (w/v) strength of benzalkonium?	$17 \times V_1 = 0.67 \times 500$ $V_1 = \dfrac{0.67 \times 500}{17}$ = 19.7 mL
Q355. Rx Ephedrine sulphate 1% e= 0.20 Chlorbutanol ½ % e= 0.18 Purified water ad 125 mL You have on hand an isotonic buffers solution pH 6.5. How many milliliters of buffered solution should be used in compounding the above preparation so that it becomes isotonic with blood plasma in order to be used as nasal drops? e = Sodium chloride equivalent	Amount of ephedrine HCl = 1/100 x 125 = 1.25 g which is equivalent to 1.25 x 0.20 =0.25g NaCl Amount of Chlorbutanol = 0.5/100 x 125 = 0.625g which is equivalent to 0.625 x 0.18 = 0.1125g NaCl Total amount of NaCl represented in the formula = 0.25 + 0.1125 = 0.3625 g NaCl. To dissolve this amount in order to make an isotonic solution, how much water is needed? $\dfrac{0.3625}{Y\,mL} \times 100 = 0.9$ $Y = \dfrac{0.3625 \times 100}{0.9}$ Y = 40.28 mL. Thus we need <u>40.28 mL. Water</u> and (125-40.28) mL. Of buffer, or <u>84.72 mL, of buffer solution</u>
Q356. How many grams of potassium citrate ($C_6H_5K_3O_7$-H_2O-mol wt 324) should be used in preparing one liter of potassium ion elixir so as to supply 15 mEq of K^+ in each 10 mL dose?	The amount of Potassium citrate containing 1 mEq of K^+ = 324/3 = 108 mg Each 10 mL contain 15 mEq, thus 1 liter should have 15 x 1000/10 = 1500 mEq. But 108mg supply 1 mEq Thus the amount required to supply 1500 mEq = 108 x 1500 = 162000 mg or 162 grams. Of Potassium citrate.
Q357. One liter of each of the belladonna extracts containing 1.15%, 1.30%, 1.35% and 1.20% of alkaloids respectively were mixed with one liter of pure solvent. What was the resulting volume and the percentage of the resulting mixture?	Using allegation medial, 1 x 1.15 = 1.15 1 x 1.30 = 1.30 1 x 1.35 = 1.35 1 x 1.20 = 1.20 <u>1 x 0 (water) = 0</u> Total 5 5 Total volume = 5 liters Concentration = 5/5 = 1% Answer.

Q358. Wool fat absorbs twice its weight of water. How much additional water will be absorbed by 5 kg hydrous wool fat containing 25% of water?	5 kg containing 25% water means there 1250 g of water and 3250g of pure wool fat.
	3250 g of pure wool fat can absorb 3250 x2 g of water
	                                                  = 6500 g water
	Thus wool fat can still absorb 6500-1250 water
	                                                  = 5250 g water. Answer

Q359. Find the amount of sodium chloride to be included in 0.5 liter of a 0.3% solution of zinc sulphate so that, on dilution with an equal quantity of water, it will be isotonic. (1% $ZnSO_4$ freezes at –0.086 °C and 1% NaCl freezes at –0.576, Plasma freezes at -0.52°C)	**Method 1:** Make a solution with twice the freezing point of plasma so that upon dilution with equal quantity of water it will have the same freezing point as plasma. Percentage of adjusting substance = $\dfrac{(2 \times 0.52) - a}{b}$

	$\% \, NaCl \, required = \dfrac{1.04 - (0.3 \times 0.086)}{0.576}$
	$= 1.76\%$ Therefore in 100 mL there will be 1.76 g **Method 2** Base the calculation on the diluted solution, i.e. instead of 100 mL of 0.3 %., calculate the amount in 200 mL of a 0.15% solution: $\dfrac{0.52 - (0.15 \times 0.086)}{0.576} = 0.88\%$ 0.88% of 200 mL has 1.76 g **Method 3:** Calculate In the normal way, ignoring the dilution. Then add contents of 100 mL of 0.9% (i.e. add 0.9 g NaCl): $\dfrac{0.52 - (0.3 \times 0.086)}{0.576} = 0.86\%$ 0.86 % of 100 ml = 086g 0.86g + 0.9 g = 1.76g
Q360. A vial of Penicillin G has 200,000 units of Pen G. Explain how you would prepare 10mL of Pen G with a concentration of 15,000 units/mL.	Total units required in 10 mL = 15,000 units/mL x 10mL = 150,000 units But the vial has 200,000 units. Thus the proportion of the required units = $\dfrac{150,000}{200,000} = \dfrac{3}{4}$ of the vial contents Therefore dissolve the dry powder in 4 mL water for injection, and use 3 mL of this reconstituted solution (which contains 150,000 units), dilute to 10 mL using water for injection aseptically.
Q361. A patient receives 500 mL I.V. drip containing 45% sodium chloride and 20,000 units of heparin sodium at a rate of 15 drops per mL. a) How many mL per hour must be administered to achieve a rate of 1200 units of heparin sodium per hour? b) How many drops per minutes should be administered?	a) 20,000 units are in 500 mL. 1200 units are in how many mL?: $\dfrac{20,000 \, units}{1200 \, units} = \dfrac{500 \, mL}{x \, mL}$ $= 30 \, mL \, per \, hour$ b) Use the formula to calculate the number of drops per minute: $R = \dfrac{V \times D}{T} \quad R = \dfrac{30 \times 15}{60} = 7.5 \, gtt/min$
Q362. Polymixin B sulphate injection contains 50,000 units of dry powder. The directions on the vial read: "Add 9.4 mL water for injection to achieve a concentration of 5000 units per mL" How many mL of the injection are needed to make the following solution?:	Amount of Polymixin B needed = 2500 units/mL x 15 mL = 37,500 units The reconstituted injection contains 5000 units per mL How many mL shall provide 37,500 units? $\dfrac{5000}{1mL} = \dfrac{37500}{XmL} \quad X = 7.5 \, mL$ Take 7.5 mL of the reconstituted solution and dilute

Polymixin B sulphate 2500 units/mL Water for inj. ad 15 mL	with water for injection to 15 mL. Answer.
Q363. An IV solution contains 40 mEq of potassium chloride in ½ L. How many mg of potassium chloride are in 750 mL? (Mol wt of KCl = 74.5)	$Wt\ of\ KCL\ containing\ 1\ mEq = \frac{Mol\ wt}{valence} = \frac{74.5}{1} = 74.5\ mg$ $40\ mEq = 40 \times 74.5 = 2980\ mg$ If 500 mL contain 2980 mg, how many mg are in 750 mL? $2980 \times \frac{750}{500} = 4470\ mg.\ Answer.$
Q364. How many calories are represented by 500 ml solution containing 10% dextrose, 9% proteins and 8% fats?	$Dextrose:\ 500 \times \frac{10}{100} \times 3.4 = 170\ kcal$ $Proteins:\ 500 \times \frac{8.5}{100} \times 4.1 = 174.25\ kcal$ $Fats:\ 500 \times \frac{9}{100} \times 9\ \ \ = \underline{405\ kcal}$ $Total =\ 749.25\ kcal.\ Answer.$
Q365. A TPN solution contains 1L of 25% dextrose, and 0.5L of 8.5% amino acid solution. Calculate its calorie: nitrogen ratio (Cal/N)	$Energy\ from\ dextrose = 1000 \times \frac{25}{100} \times 3.4 = 850\ kcal$ $Amount\ of\ amino\ acids = 500\ mL \times \frac{8.5}{100} = 42.5\ g$ $Amount\ of\ Nitrogen = \frac{42.5}{6.25} = 6.8$ $Calorie:\ Nitrogen\ ratio = 850:6.8 = \ \ \ 125:1\ \ \ Answer.$
Q366. 1500 mL of a TPN solution contains 5% dextrose and 4.25% amino acids. What is the protein-calorie percentage of the solution?	$Calories\ from\ dextrose:\ 1500 \times \frac{5}{100} \times 3.4 = 255\ kcal$ $Calories\ from\ amino\ acid:\ 1500 \times \frac{4.25}{100} \times 4.1 = 261.4\ kcal$ $Total\ calories = 255 + 261.4 = 516.4$ $Protein\text{-}calorie\ percentage = \frac{261.4}{516.4} \times 100 = 50.6\%\ Answer.$

Chapter 17 Practice questions

QUESTIONS	Answers
Q1p. Givet interprétations of the following prescriptions : a. M. et ft ung. Disp. 10g b. Caps I. q.i.f. p.c. et h.s. c. M. et ft. sol. 1g/tbsp d. Propranolol HCl 5 mg p.o. t.id a.c. &h.s e. Gtt. IV ad. m. & n. f. M. et ft. inj. For I.V. use.	
Q2p. Complete the following a. 0.50.25 mg = ...g = ...kg = ... µg b. 5000 µg = ...mg = ...ng = ...pg c. 0.0075 kg = ... g = ... µg = ...mg d. 0.005 L = ...mL = ... mL = ... µL e. 440 mL = ...L = ... µL = ... GL f. Adhesive tape made from a polyvinyl fabric has tensile strength 25.45 kg per 2.55 cm. Reduce these quantities to g per mm. g. Reduce 25.500 g to µg, mg and to kg. h. Analytical Instrument A can detect presence of a drug in nanogram, while Instrument B can detect the same drug down to pictogram. How many more capable is Instrument A compared to Instrument B? i. I have upgraded the hard disc of my computer from 80 megabytes to 10 Gigabytes. What is the increased capacity in megabytes?	
Q3p. Fill in the blanks: a. 1. 1,900 kg + 453 g + 65000mg =...............g b. 60 mg+70000 mcg + 250,000 ng =............mcg c. 2. 453cm + 8.55 m + 78000mm = ... cm d. 320 mL + 5.22 m + 45,000mm = ...cm e. 3. 0.75m + 2200 cm + 0. 75 cm = ...m f. 6.45 L + 65 mL + 7000 µL = ...mL	
Q4p. A 500mg tablet has A, B, and C ingredients. The amount of A and B is 0.05g and 240 mg respectively. What is the weight of ingredient C?	
Q5p. The following weights were removed from a container, originally containing 1.5 kg: : 22g, 435 g, 202.4 g and 45.5 g. How much was left in the container?	
Q6p. You are asked to prepare acetylsalicylic acid tablets each of which to contain 75 mg of the active ingredient. How much acetylsalicylic acid do you need to prepare 300 tablets?	
Q7p. Multiply 230 mg by 64, divide the results by 115 and reduce the results to grams.	

Q8p. A patient has been prescribed 250 nanograms alfacalcidol tablets to be taken twice a day for thirty days. How many mg does the patient receive in 30 days?	
Q9p. 50 mL peppermint oil was used to manufacture 20,000 capsules. Calculate the amount of peppermint oil in each capsule and express your answer in microliters.	
Q10p. Microgynon 30® contains levonogestrel 150 micrograms and ethynyl estradiol 30 micrograms. How many grams of each ingredient would be used in making 10,000 tablets?	
Q11p. A dose of Qvar®, an aerosol inhaler, contains 50 µg of beclomethasone dipropionate per inhalation dose. There are usually 200 doses. What is the total amount of beclomethasone in the inhaler?	
Q12p. An Ergortamine suppository contains the following ingredients: Ergotamine Tartarate 2.0 mg Caffeine 0.1 g Cocoa Butter q.s ad 3.0 g a. Calculate the amount of cocoa butter required in this prescription. b. How much Ergortamine is required to make 30 suppositories?	

Q13p.
    Rx Isoniazid   1.0 g
        Citric acid monohydrate   0.25 g
        Sodium citrate   1.2 g
        concentrated anis water   1.0 mL
        Compound tatrazine solution 1.0 mL
        Glycerol   1.0 mL
Chloroform water, double strength   40 mL
Purified water,
freshly boiled and cooled to   100 mL
 	
Sig 5mL bid for 1/12
 	
    a. How many mL of this prescription would you make?
    b. How many kg of isoniazid would you need?
    c. How many L of Chloroform water is needed?
    d. How much water is needed?
	a) 300 mL
	b) 0.3 kg
	c) 0.12 L
	d) 171 mL

Q14p. An intravenous solution of Metronidazole contains 5 mg/mL. If 200 mL of this solution is mixed with 0.48 L of Normal saline infusion,
    a. What is the concentration in mcg/mL of metronidazole in the infusion?
    b. If the infusion is given for a period of one hour, how many milligrams of metronidazole does the patient get per minute?
	a). 1471mcg/mL
	
	b)16.67 mg/min

Q15p. 2000µg of a drug were added to 750 mL of Dextrose –Saline infusion. How	675 mL

many mL of this infusion would contain 1.8 mg of the drug.	

Q16p. An anthelminthic piperazine citrate Elixir PCx contains the following ingredients:
    Piperazine citrate   18.75 g
    Peppermint spirit   0.5 mL
    Green s and Tatrazine solution 1.5 mL
    Glycerol   20 mL
    Syrup   50 mL
    Purified water ,
    freshly boiled and cooled *to* 100 mL
 	
a. The dose of an 8 year old child is 750 mg. How many mL of the drug should be given to this child?
b. If we were to make 40 mL only of piperazine citrate elixir, how much of piperazine citrate would we need?
	a) 4 mL
	
	b) 7.5 g

Q17p. a) A vial of Lasix® injection contains 10mg/mL of frusemide. How many micrograms of frusemide would be contained in 0.5mL of the injection? b) You have been asked to prepare anti-cold tablets containing the following active ingredients: Chlorpheniramine maleate ....2 mg Paracetamol ....250 mg Pseudoephedrine HCl ....30 mg Dextromethorphan HCl ....15mg Caffeine .... 100 mg i) If you have 1 kg of paracetamol powder, how many tablets can you make? ii) From the tablets you have made in (a), how many grams of the rest of the ingredients would you need?	a) 5000 mcg b) (i) 4000 tablets ii) Chlorpheniramine 8.0 g Pseudoephedrine 120.0 g Dextromethorphan 60 g Caffeine 400 g
Q18p. Convert the following: 34 mL = ...fl oz. = ... pt f ℨii ss = ...♏ = ...μL 50 L = ...gal = ...fl oz 880 mL = ...pt = ...fl oz 0.2 L = ...♏ =................ fℨ 15 pt = ... L =..... ....fℨ 1 gal 3 pt = ...mL = ...μL 4 gal 2 pt 6 fl oz = ...mL = ...L 300 pt = ... f ℨ= .... mL 45 kg = ...lb = ... oz 769000 mg = ...gr = ...oz 153.78 g = ... oz =................lb 681g = ...lb =...............oz 452 lb = ...g =................Kg 15 gr = ...mg = ...mcg 12 in = ... cm = ...km 0.25 km = ...in = ...cm	

Q19p. The tensile strength of an adhesive tape is 3kg/1.27 cm. Express this in terms of lb / in.	6.6/2.23 lb./in
Q20p. The diameter of oil globules in an emulsion is 2 μm. What is this size in inches	7.9×10^{-5} inches
Q21p. Digoxin was infused at 0.75 mg per hour. Express this rate in ng/minute.	12,500 ng/minute
Q22p. You are asked to prepare 42 capsules of atropine sulphate, each of which containing 1/250 gr. You do not have atropine sulphate powder, but you have 400 mcg atropine sulphate tablets in your store. How many of these tablets would you need?	28 tablets
Q23p. a) The cost of adrenaline is 5,000 shillings per 100 g. How much would it cost to prepare 50 tablets each having 2 ½ gr adrenalin? b) Anti-anemia tablet contain 525 mg ferrous sulphate, equivalent to 105 mg elemental iron. If a patient has a prescription calling for Ferrous sulphate tablets I tds x 4/52, how many grains of elemental iron would the patient get?	a) 405 Shs. b) 135.7 gr
Q24p. The dose of quinine is 5-10 mg per kg body weight. Express this dose in terms of gr/lb. body weight.	0.035 – 0.7 gr/lb.
Q25p. How many milligrams are present in a 1/150 gr Nitrostat tablet?	0.43mg
Q26p. How many 1/200 gr of tablets can be prepared from 500 mg of active ingredient?	1538 tablets
Q27p. How many milligrams of Guiafenesin will be present in 480mL (15 mg/5 mL) of solution?	1440 mg
Q28p. If the retail cost of each Zyprexa tablet is TShs 3800, what would be the retail cost for 30 tablets?	Shs 114,000.00
Q29p. How many grams of dextrose are required to prepare a 1000 mL D5W solution?	50 g
Q30p. How much atropine is required to prepare a 1:500, 500 mL solution of atropine ?	1 g
Q31p. How many grams of Lignocaine are required to dispense 1 quart of 1 in 50 solution?	19.2 g
Q32p. How many calories are provided by 1 quart of a 1 in 500 solution of dextrose?	163.2 Cal
Q33p. How much Xylocaine is required to prepare 30 mL of a 1:500 solution of Xylocaine?	0.06 g
Q34p. In what proportion should 49% alcohol be mixed with water to prepare 1000 mL of a 25% alcohol solution?	24:25
Q35p. How much Heparin is required to dispense a 0.25% 750 mL solution?	1.875 g
Q36p. If a prescription calls for "Biaxin 500 mg p.o. bid x 10 days", how many mL of Biaxin 125 mg/5 mL are required to dispense a 10-day supply?	400 mL
Q37p. If a prescription is written to take 50 mg of diphenhydramine by mouth four times a day for 5 days, how many mL of 12.5 mg/5 mL diphenhydramine solution are required to dispense 5 day supply?	4000 mL
Q38p. If 125 mcg of a drug are diluted with water up to 50 mL, what is the % of drug ?	0.0025%
Q39p. If 1 tablespoonful of Thioridazine intense solution (100 mg/mL) is diluted with water up to 1 quart, what is the % of drug in the final solution?	0.15625%
Q40p. If 10 teaspoonfuls of Risperdal oral solution (100 mcg/5 mL) are diluted	2.08 mcg/mL

with water up to 480 mL, what is the concentration of drug in mcg/mL in the final solution?	
Q41p. How many mL of 10% Benzoyl peroxide are required to prepare 20 mL of 5% Benzoyl peroxide solution?	10 mL
Q42p. How many milligrams of Clindamycin are present in 60 mL of 0.1% topical gel of clindamycin?	60 mg
Q43p. How many tablets of 250 mg erythromycin are required to prepare 500 mL of 2%. topical solution of erythromycin?	40 tablets
Q44p. If 325 mg of ferrous sulfate contains 22% elementary iron, how many milligrams of elemental iron will the patient receive with each dose of 325 mg iron?	71.5 mg
Q45p. If niferex liquid solution provides 10 mg of elemental iron in 1 teaspoonful, how many mL of solution are required to provide 55 mg of elemental iron ?	27.5 mL
Q46p. If 3 capsules of 150 mg of Clindamycin are added to 150 mL of 1% Cleocin topical solution, what is the % of Clindamycin in the final mixture	1.3%
Q47p. How many grams of Heparin are required to prepare 1 quart of 0.45% solution?	4.32 g
Q48p. How many grams of Dextrose are required to prepare 5% of 500 mL solution?	25g
Q49p. How many 500 mg tablets of erythromycin are required to prepare 240 mL of 2% solution of erythromycin?	10 tablets
Q50p. How many milligrams are equal to 1/150 gr of Nitroglycerine?	0.43 mg
Q51p. How much Atropine is required to dispense 1 quart of 1 in 100 solution?	9600 mg
Q52p. If 60 mg of elementary iron are present in 325 mg of ferrous sulfate, what is the % of elementary iron?	18.46%
Q53p. How much Lignocaine is required to prepare 1 : 1000, 30 mL of solution of Lignocaine?	30 mg
Q54p. If 60 gm of 1% hydrocortisone are mixed with 80 gm of 2.5% hydrocortisone, what is the % of hydrocortisone in the final mixture?	1.85%
Q55p. If a prescription reads "Augmentin 875 mg by mouth twice a day", how many mL of Augmentin 400 mg/5 mL are required to dispense a 10 day supply?	218.75 mL
Q56p. How many mL of 75% alcohol should be mixed with 10% of 1000 mL alcohol to prepare 30% of 500 mL alcohol solution ?	153.84 mL
Q57p. If a prescription reads "Augmentin 875 mg p.o. bid x 10 days," how many mL of Augmentin 250 mg/5 mL are required to fill a ten-day supply?	350 mL
Q58p. If 1000 tablets of Risperdal 1 mg cost 3.6 million shillings and the mark-up on prescription is 20%, what would be the retail price for 30 tablets?	Shs 129,600
Q59p. How many 975 mg tablets of aspirin are required to prepare 100 tablets of 75 mg?	6 tablets
Q60p. If 1 teaspoonful of Thioridazine concentrated solution (30 mg/mL) is diluted up to the 480 mL mark with plain water, what is the strength of drug in mg/mL in the final solution?	0.31mg/mL
Q61p. If a prescription reads "Diphenhydramine 50 mg p.o. hs x 30 days",	600 mL

what would be the dispensed quantity of drug in mL (12.5 mg / 5 mL) for thirty-day supply?	
Q62p. Erythromycin 60 mL of a 2% topical solution contains how many grams?	1.2g
Q63p. If 250 mg of Cefazolin powder are diluted with water up to the 250 mL mark, what is the % of drug in the final solution ?	0.1%
Q64p. A manufacturing pharmacist has three lots of ichthamol ointment, containing 50%, 25%, and 10% of ichthamol. How many grams of each may be used to prepare 4800 g of a 20% ichthamol ointment?	50% =872.73g 25% =872.73g 10% = 3054.55g
Q65. If a prescription reads "100 mcg cyanocobalamin i.m. every week", how many ampoules of 1000 mcg / mL are required to fill a month supply?	1 ampoule
Q66. You are directed to prepare 10 liters of a 1:5000 solution of potassium permanganate. If the potassium permanganate is available only in the form of tablets, each containing 0.2 g, how many tablets should be used in preparing the solution?	10 tablets
Q67p. How much Clobetasole is present in 60 gm of 0.5% ointment?	0.3 g
Q68p. Find out the weight in gm of 500 mL glycerin [Specific gravity = 1.25 gm/mL]	625 g
Q69pFind out the volume of 5 lb. of glycerin. [density = 1.25 gm/mL]	1816 mL
Q70p. Calculate the weight of 500 mL of acid. [density of acid = 2.5 gm/mL]	1250 g
Q71p. The adult dose of a drug is 500 mg. What is the dose for a 2 year old child? [use young rule]	11.56
Q72p. The adult dose of a drug is 750 mg, what is the dose for child weighing 20 lbs.?	100mg
Q73p. If a dropper is calibrated to deliver 325 mg of iron sulfate in 0.6 mL and an adult dose of drug is 325 mg, what is the dose of a drug in mL for a 15 month old infant?	0.06 mL
Q74p. If an adult dose of a drug is 100 mg, what would be the dose for a child having a body surface area of 20 mm$_2$?	11.56 mg
Q75p. How many milligrams are in 10 grains of aspirin?	650 mg
Q76p. If a normal dose of a drug is 10 mg/kg/day, how many 250 mg/100mL ready-infusion bags are required to fill the above order for a 70kg Patient.	3 bags
Q77p. If the prescription calls for "50 micrograms of a drug three times daily for 10 days", how many 1/100 grain tablets are required to fill the above order ?	3 tabs
Q78p. If a prescription reads "Lanoxin 0.125 mg by mouth every day", how many mL of Lanoxin 50 mcg/mL are required to dispense a 30 day supply?	75 mL
Q79p. If a prescription reads to dissolve 2 gm of guaifenesin in 100 mL of water, how many grains of guaifenesin are present in 1 teaspoonful of solution	1.53 gr
Q80p. If 100 mg of Lactin is equal to 4500 units, how many milligrams are required to obtain 1 unit?	0.02 mg
Q81p. f a prescription reads "Ampicillin 50 mg by mouth twice a day" for a 7 year old child, how many mL (125 mg/5 mL) are required to dispense a 7 day supply of the drug?	28 mL
Q82p. What is the dose of a drug for a person having 110 m$_2$ body surface area? The average adult dose of the drug is 750 mg.	477 mg

Q83p. How many grams of a drug are required to prepare 240 mL of 10% solution?	24 g
Q84p. How many grams of sodium chloride are required to make 750 mL of 0.9% normal saline solution?	6.75 g
Q85p. How many grams of dextrose are present in 500 mL of $D_{25}W$ solution?	125 g
Q86p. How much Povidone-Iodine is required to prepare 1000 mL of 1 in 750 solution?	1.33g
Q87p. How much Lignocaine is required to prepare 30 mL of 1:1000 solution?	30 mg
Q88p. How many grams of dextrose are needed to prepare 5L of 1 in 250 solution?	20g
Q89p. What is the % of boric acid in 1 in 20 solution?	5%
Q90p. To dispense 5% of 250 mL solution of Thioridazine, how many mL of 30 mg/mL are required?	417 mL
Q91p. If 20 mL of Risperdal 1mg/mL are diluted with water up to 240 mL mark, what would be the strength of drug in mg /mL?	0.08 mg/mL
Q92p. How much dextrose is required to prepare 1 in 100, 50 mL dextrose solution?	0.5g
Q93p. How many Milliequivalent of sodium are present in a 5% 1-pint sodium bicarbonate solution? [MW = 84 gm/mole]	285.71 mEq
Q94p. If the recommended dose of a drug is 0.01 mcg/kg four times weekly, approximately how many ampoules (2mcg/ mL) are required to fill a week supply? (Patient's weight = 110 lbs.)	1 ampule.
Q95p. If the recommended dose of Reclast (5mg/mL) is 0.25 mcg/kg/min, how long will it take to finish up 2.5mg/mL? (Patient's weight = 110 lbs.)	200 min
Q96p. Five packs of K-Lor powder (each pack = 8mEq of KCl) should dissolve in 12oz of water. If 5mL of this resultant solution is diluted up to the 25mL mark with plain water, what would be the final concentration of KCl in mg/mL? (K = 39, Cl = 35.5). (oz. = 30mL)	1.66 mg/mL
Q97p. Kaletra Oral solution, an antiretroviral drug contains lopinavir 100 mg and ritonavir 25 mg in each 5 mL. If a prescription reads 400mg of Ritonavir daily, how many mL of Kaletra (100mg/25mg per 5 mL) oral solution are required to fill a 7-day supply?	140 mL
Q98p. If 1mL of Ensure provides 1 calorie, how many ounces of Ensure are required to provide 0.1Kcal?	3.3 oz.
Q99p. How many milligrams of Atenolol is present in each mL of a 0.015% eye drop?	0.15mg/mL
Q100p. Floxin eye drops are available as a 0.0002% ophthalmic solution. How many milligrams of drug is present in each mL of solution?	0.002mg/mL
Q101p. The recommended dose of Rhinocort aqua nasal spray is 32mcg daily as one spray per nostril. If nasal spray provides 40 sprays (each with 16mcg) after initial priming, how many days will this nasal spray last?	19 days
Q102p. If the standard infusion rate of Primacor is 0.25mg/kg/hr., how many mL per minute will be administered to a patient weighing 110 lbs.? (Primacor 250 mL, 1 infusion bag 0.2 mg/mL)	1 mL/Min
Q103p. A digoxin potency in elixir dosage form is 80% compared to digoxin I.V. dosage formulations. If a prescription says 5mL (25mcg/ mL) per day,	121.6 mcg I.V == 125 mcg oral

what would be an equivalent dose of the drug in milligrams for I.V. dosage form?	
Q104p. If 6.5 g of glycerol, having a specific gravity 1.25, was dissolved in 21 mL water. What would be the % strength expressed in w/v, w/w, and v/v?	24.8%w/v 23.6 w/w 19.85 v/v
Q105p. Sulfur 3% Salicylic acid 3% White Petrolatum.............q.s. 80 gm Find out the amount of Sulfur required to fill the above prescription?	2.4 g

Q106p.
Rx
    a. Codeine phosphate 920 mg
    b. Robitussin® syrup 30 mL
    c. Elixophylline ad   240 mL
If a dropper delivers 20 drops per mL, and the dose of codeine phosphate is 0.5 mg/kg body weight, How many drops of the prescription should be administered as a dose to a 22-lb child?
	26 drops

Q108p. A certain liniment is prepared by mixing 2 lb. of methyl salicylate (sp. gr. 1.18), 1 liter of alcohol (sp. gr. 0.8) and 1 lb. of chloroform (sp. gr. 1.475). What is the volume, in milliliters, of the mixture?	2376

Q109p.
Rx
    Clindamycin Hydrochloride 0.6 g
    Propylene Glycol 6.0 mL
    Purified water 8.0 mL
    Isopropyl alcohol ad 60.0 mL
    a. Calculate the amount of each ingredient required to prepare one liter of the solution.
    b. How many capsules, each containing 150 mg clindamycin hydrochloride, would be used to prepare the prescription.
    c. What would be the percentage concentration (w/v) of clindamycin hydrochloride in the prescription?
	a) 1 L contains 10 g Clindamycin; 100 mL Propylene glycol; and 133.3 mL water
	b) 4 capsules
	c) 1%w/v

Q110p. How many grams of silver nitrate should be used in preparing 500 mL of a solution such that 10 mL diluted to a liter will yield a 1:5000 solution?	10g

Q111p. A modified Ringer's solution has the following formula:
    Sodium chloride 8.60 g
    Potassium chloride 0.30 g
    Calcium chloride 0.33 g
    PEG 3350 60.00 g
    Water for injection ad   1000.00 mL
Assuming that 980 mL of water are used in preparing the solution, calculate the specific gravity of the solution.
	s.g. =1.0492

Q112p. A Cough mixture oral solution 250 mg/5 mL.
    Sig. tablespoon t.i.d. for 10d
    (a) How many milliliters of medicine should be dispensed?
    (b) How many total milligrams of medicine are contained in the final volume?
	a) 450 mL
	b) 22500 mg
	c) 9 bottles

(c) How many bottles will be dispensed to a patient who takes two tablespoonful of the medicine? (each bottle is 100 mL)		
Q113p. Rx Potassium permanganate q.s. Purified water ad 500 mL Sig. Two teaspoons diluted to a liter equals a 1:5000 solution. How many 0.4g tablets of potassium permanganate should be used in compounding the prescription?	25 tablets	
Q114p. A prescription calls for 1000mL of an IV infusion to be administered over a 6 hours period. How many drops per min should be delivered to the patient, by using an IV administration set that delivers 8 drops per mL?	22 drops	

Q115p. Rx   Zephiran Chloride Solution (17% w/v)   q.s.
    Purified water, to make   480 mL
    Sig. One tbsp. diluted to 1 gallon with water to make a 1:10,000 dilution
How many milliliters of zephiran chloride solution should be used to in preparing the prescription?
	71.247 mL	

Q116p. Given that an average BSA of an adult is 1.73 m^2. The usual pediatric dose of cefazolin sodium is 50mg/kg day divided equally into three doses, what would be one dose in milligram for a child weighing 33 1b?	250 mg	
Q117p. An industrial pharmacist wishes to prepare a drug solution, how may grams of potassium permanganate should be used in preparing 50mL of a solution such that two tablespoonful diluted to half a liter will yield a 1:800 solution.	1.04 g	
Q118p. If an intravenous solution contain 123mg of a drug substance in each 250mL bottle is to be administered at the rate of 200mg of drug per minute, how many milliliters of the solution would be given per hour?	24.39 mL	
Q119p. The child dose of a drug is 40mg/kg/day. If a child was given a daily dose of 2 teaspoonfuls of the drug suspension containing 140mg of a drug per 5mL, what was the weight in pound, of the child?	15.4 lb.	

Q120p. A cold tablet contains the following amounts of active ingredients:
    Acetaminophen   325mg
    Chlorpheniramine maleate   2mg
    Pseudoephedrine HCl   30mg
    Dextromethorphan HCl 15mg
How many tablets may be prepared if a manufacturing pharmacist has 1kg of acetaminophen, 125g of chlorpheniramine maleate, and unlimited quantities of the other two ingredients?
	3076 tablets	

Q121p. A pharmacist failed to place the balance in equilibrium before weighing 200mg of the drug. Later, he discovered that the balance was out of equilibrium and that a 20% error was incurred. If the balance pan on which he placed the drug was light, how many milligrams of the drug did he actually weigh?	160 g	
Q122p. The child dose of a drug is 40mg/kg/day. If a child was given a daily dose of 2 tablespoonfuls of the drug suspension containing 140mg of a drug per 5mL, what was the weight in pound, of the child?	46.2 lb.	

Q123p.
    Rx   Paregoric   15.0 mL
    Pectin   0.6 g
    Kaolin   22.0 g
    Alcohol   0.8 mL
    Purified water   ad   120.0 mL
	a) 0.625mL
	b) 150 mg
	c) 200 µl	

Mix and make a suspension. Sig. two tablespoon p.r.n. for diarrhea. How many mL of paregoric would be contained in each teaspoon dose? How many mg of pectin would be contained in each prescribed dose? How many mcL of alcohol would be contained in each dose?	
Q124p. If a medication order calls for 720 mL of DNS infusion to be administered to a 154-1b patient over a period of 2 hours. Using an Intravenous administration set that delivers 10 drops/mL. How many drops per second should be delivered to a 110-1b patients	1 drop/sec

Q125p.
The following regimen of oral prednisolone is prescribed for a patient:
    50 mg/d x   10 days; then
    25 mg/d x 10 day; then
    12.5 mg/d x 10 days; then
    5 mg/d x 10 days; and then
    5 mg/d x 10 weeks.
How many scored 25-mg tablets and how many 5-mg tablets should be dispensed to meet the dosing requirements?
	35 25mg tablets
	80 5mg tablets

Q126p. In each of the following express the answer in grams.
    Add 0.5kg, 50mg, and 2.5g. Reduce the result to grams.
    Add 0.00250kg, 1750mg, 2.25g and 825,000mg.
	a) 502.55 g
	b) 831.50 g

Q127p. A pharmacist weighed 825mg of a drug, when checked on another balance, the weight was found to be 805mg. Calculate the deviation from the second weighing in terms of percentage.	3.03%
Q128p. How may drops would be prescribed in each dose of a 110-1b person, of a liquid medicine if 30mL contain 60 doses? The dispensing dropper calibrates 20 drops per milliliter (given 1 Lt equals to 1,000mL).	10 drops

Q129p.
Rx Hydrocodone Bitartrate   0.2 g
    Phenacetin   3.6 g
    Aspirin   6.0 g
    Caffeine   0.6 g
    M. ft. caps. no. xxxvi
    Sig. ii caps. t.i.d. p.r.n. for pain
 	
How many milligrams of Hydrocodone bitartrate would be contained in each capsule?
What is the total weight in milligrams of the ingredients in each capsule?
How many milligrams of caffeine would be taken daily.
	a) 5.9 mg
	
	b) 105.9 mg phenacetin
	
	c) 176.5 g Aspirin
	
	d) 17.65 g Caffeine

Q130p.
    ℞Coal Tar   50g
    Bentonite   80 g
    Water   300 mL
    Hydrophilic ointment   80g
    Zinc oxide, to make   1000g
	Coal tar 227.5g
	Bentonite 364 g
	Water 1365 mL
	Hydrophilic
	    Ung. 364 g
	ZnO to 4550 g

	How much of each ingredient should be used in preparing 10-1b of the ointment?	

Q131p.
Rx Erythromycin Estolate 400 mg/5mL
Disp. 100mL
Sig._____ tsp. q.i.d. until all medication is take.
 	
If the dose of erythromycin estolate is given as 40 mg/kg per day.
   a) What would be the proper dose of the medication in the Signa if the prescription is for a 44-1b child?
   b) How many days will the medication last?
		a) 2.5 mL (1/2 teaspoon) 4 times a day
		
		b) 10 days

Q132p. The usual dose of digoxin for rapid digitalization is a total of 1.0 mg. divided into two or more portions at intervals of 6 to 8 hours. How many milliliters of digoxin elixir containing 50µg/mL would provide this dose?		20 mL daily, 10 mL bd 6.7 mL tid 5 mL qid
Q133p. The dose of beclomethasone, an aerosolized inhalant, is 200 µg twice daily. The commercial inhaler delivers 50 µg per metered inhalation and contains 200 inhalations. How many inhalers should be dispensed to a patient if a 60-day supply is prescribed?		3 inhalers
Q134p. Rx Piperazine syrup 500mg/5mL Disp. _____ mL Sig. Parents: Take ____ teaspoonful daily for 2 days Child: Take ____ teaspoonfuls daily for 2 days. The dose of piperazine for adults is 3.5 g as a single daily dose for 2 consecutive days. For children, the dose is 75 mg/kg of body weight per day for 2 consecutive days. If both parents and a 66-1b child are to take the medication as directed, How many milliliters of piperazine syrup should be dispensed? How many teaspoonfuls each should the parents and the child take daily?		185 mL piperazine Parents: 7 teaspoons daily Child: 4 ½ tsp daily
Q135p. How may milliliters each of phenytoin sodium suspensions containing 30 mg per 5mL and 125 mg per 5mL should be used in preparing 480mL of a suspension containing 10mg of phenytoin sodium per milliliter?		125mg/5mL: 101 mL 30 mg/5 mL: 379 mL
Q136p. Convert 30°C and 100°C into °F		86°F; 212°F
Q137p. Convert 120°F and 77°F into °C		48.9°C; 15°C
Q138p. Calculate the flow rate of an IV infusion in gtt/min to administer 400 mL for 8 hrs if the infusion set is calibrated at the drop factor of 15 gtt/mL.		13 gtt/min
Q139p. The label on Penicillin G package reads: **Penicillin G Potassium (buffered)** (5,000,000 Units) Add 23 mL sterile water to make a solution 200,000 units/mL		Add 8 mL sterile water to the penicillin pack.

How many mL of sterile water for injection should be used to prepare the following solution?: Pen G Potassium (buffered) 5,000,000 units Sterile water for injection q.s. Make solution containing 500,000 units/mL Sig: "One mL = 500,000 units of Pen G Potassium" Hint: Calculate the volume occupied by dry powder. Then if you use 23 mL sterile water the resulting solution is 200,000 units/mL. How many mL should be used to obtain 500,000 units/mL?	
Q140p. Two units of blood, 500mL each are to be infused for 4 hours. If the infusion is calibrated at 15 drops per mL, calculate the IV flow rate in gtt/min.	63 gtt/min
Q141p. Alfentany HCl, an anesthetic drug, is administered at the rate of 2.2µg/kg/min to induce anesthesia. How long will the infusion take to administer 0.55 mg to a 75 kg patient	3.3 min
Q142p. A 152lb patient was prescribed Insulin suspension at the dose of 1 unit/kg/24hr. How many units of isophane insulin should be administered daily?	69 units
Q143p. In children, Heparin is administered in the dose of 60 units/kg - 80 units/kg every 4 hours. Express this range in terms of mL/day of heparin injection containing 5000 units/mL for a 25 kg child.	1.8 mL/day-2.4 mL/day
Q144p. An IV infusion for a 25 kg child is to contain 17.5 mg of Vancomycin HCl per kg bd wt in 200 mL NS. You have on hand a 7.5 mL vial containing 500 mg dry vancomycin powder. How would you obtain the needed amount on vancomycin for the infusion?	Use 6.6 mL from the vial.
Q145p. 1.5 L of 0.5% potassium chloride infusion solution is to be administered to a patient. How many mEq are represented in the infusion?	100.7 mEq
Q146p. How many mL of Ammonium chloride solution (100 mEq/10 mL) should be added to ½ L of D5W which is to be administered to a 50-kg patient who requires 0.3 mEq per Kg body wt?	1.4 mL
Q147p What is the osmolarity of a solution containing 10% dextrose? (Mo wt of Dextrose =180)	556 mOsmol/L
Q148p. Express the concentration of 2.94% calcium chloride solution as mOsmol/L, assuming 100% dissociation (Mol wt of $CaCl_2.2H_2O$ = 147)	60 mOsmol/L
Q149p. Calculate the ratio of Caloric:Nitrogen ratio of a TPN solution consisting of 1 L of 10% dextrose and 0.75 L of 4.25% amino acid solution	113:1
Q150p. Calculate the protein-calorie percentage of a liter of 10% dextrose containing 8.5% amino acids	50.6%
Q151p. What is the pH of a buffer solution prepared with 0.05M sodium borate and 0.005M boric acid? (the pKa value of boric acid is 9.29 at 25°C	10.24 Answer.
Q152p. What would be total calories provided by TPN mixture containing 1200mL D5W,1000 mL of 10% amino acids, 100 mL of 5% alcohol and 300 mL of 20% fat emulsion ?	1189.6 kcal
Q153p. If an I.V. admixture contains 1000mg of drug in 250 mL solution, how	250 drops/min

| many drops per minute are required to infuse 50mg of drug per minute ? [I.V set delivers 20 drops/mL] | |

APPENDIX 1

SOME EQUIVALENCES AND FORMULAE TO REMEBER

1 Kilogram	= 1000 grams	1 OZ	= 30 mL
1 Gram	= 1000 milligrams	16 OZ	= 480 mL = 1 Pint
1 Milligram	= 1000 micrograms	1 Pint	= 480 mL
1 Microgram	= 0.001 milligrams	1 Quart	= 960 mL = 2 Pints
1 Milligrams	= 0.001 grams	1 Gallon	= 3840 mL = 4 Quarts = 8 Pints
1 Microgram	= 10^{-6} grams	2.2 lbs	= 1 kg
1 Nanogram	= 10^{-9} grams	1 Teaspoonful	= 5 mL
1 Grain	= 65 milligrams	1 Tablespoonful	= 15 mL
1 Litre	= 1000 mL	1 Teacupful	= 120 mL
		1 Wineglassful	= 60 mL
		1 Tumblerful	= 240 mL

Density = Weight / volume

Proof Gallon = $\dfrac{\text{gallon x \% V/V strength}}{50\% \text{ V/V}}$

Proof Gallon = $\dfrac{\text{gallon x proof strength}}{100 \text{ proof}}$

Equivalent wt = $\dfrac{\text{gram atomic weight}}{\text{valence}}$

Milliequivalent = $\dfrac{\text{equivalent weight}}{1000}$

Young's Rule   Child dose = $\dfrac{\text{Age in year}}{\text{Age} + 12}$

Drilling's rule   Child dose = $\dfrac{\text{Age in year x adult dose}}{12}$

Fried's rule   Child dose = $\dfrac{\text{Age in month x adult dose}}{150}$

Clark's rule   Child dose = $\dfrac{\text{Weight in lb x adult dose}}{150}$

Child dose = $\dfrac{\text{Body surface area of child x adult dose}}{\text{Body surface area of adult}}$

Child dose = $\dfrac{\text{Body surface area of child x adult dose}}{173 \text{ M}^2}$

Caloric Density of Nutritional substrates:

Nutritional Substance	Caloric density (kcal/g)
Glucose, anhydrous	3.85
Glucose, hydrous	3.4
Protein	4.0
Fat Emulsion	9.0
Alcohol	7.0